Life in the Victorian Asylum

In the labourer and artificer class the lunatic is so far fortunate that, living from hand to mouth under the sweat of his brow, the outbreak of insanity generally pauperises him at once and throws the responsibility of his care and treatment upon the public authorities. The law of the land is admirably designed for his protection and welfare, and, if it be really carried out, the care and proper treatment of the pauper lunatic will be all that humanity and science can desire. He will be placed forthwith in one of the county asylums, a class of institutions of which our own profession and the community at large have every reason to be abundantly proud, and he will there receive care and treatment which his superiors in rank and wealth may well regard with jealous envy.

Excerpt from *A Manual of Psychological Medicine*,
by John Charles Bucknill and Daniel Hack Tuke, 1879.

Life in the Victorian Asylum

The World of Nineteenth Century Mental Health Care

Mark Stevens

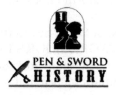

PEN & SWORD
HISTORY

First published in Great Britain in 2014 by
Pen & Sword History
an imprint of
Pen & Sword Books Ltd
47 Church Street
Barnsley
South Yorkshire
S70 2AS

ISBN 978 1 78159 373 8

A CIP catalogue record for this book is available from the British
Library

Typeset in Ehrhardt by
Mac Style, Bridlington, East Yorkshire
Printed and bound in the UK by CPI Group (UK) Ltd, Croydon,
CRO 4YY

Pen & Sword Books Ltd incorporates the imprints of Pen & Sword
Archaeology, Atlas, Aviation, Battleground, Discovery, Family
History, History, Maritime, Military, Naval, Politics, Railways,
Select,
Transport, True Crime, and Fiction, Frontline Books, Leo Cooper,
Praetorian Press, Seaforth Publishing and Wharncliffe.

For a complete list of Pen & Sword titles please contact
PEN & SWORD BOOKS LIMITED
47 Church Street, Barnsley, South Yorkshire, S70 2AS, England
E-mail: enquiries@pen-and-sword.co.uk
Website: www.pen-and-sword.co.uk

Contents

Acknowledgements

This book would not exist without the archives of Fair Mile Hospital, Cholsey (formerly known, and referred to in this book as the Moulsford Asylum). Thanks are due to John Man of the Berkshire Healthcare NHS Trust for his work in rescuing much of the archive before it could be dispersed or destroyed. Thanks are then due to Sue Crossley at The Wellcome Trust for her help in securing a grant to list and repair the archive.

In terms of publishing this book, a vast array of thanks must go to Jen Newby at Pen and Sword. Jen is always patiently solving my problems and generally being decent to me; one day I hope to repay the compliment. I must also thank my family again for putting up with the hours of extra work that writing a book entails. It is an indulgence and I always try to remember that.

I also need to thank everyone I meet at my talks who is curious of mind. You have asked questions that kept me working to understand what life was like for the patients and staff of Victorian asylums. This is like having an army of additional editors. Then there are a number of people in Cholsey who keep the memories of Fair Mile alive. I would like to single out Bill Nicholls and Ian Wheeler for their efforts.

The acknowledgements in *Broadmoor Revealed* ended with an appreciation of everyone who had been touched by a Broadmoor story. I would like to reiterate that, then add in all those people who were touched by Fair Mile and the other Victorian asylums up and down the country. Whatever your experiences, you will never be forgotten.

Preface

I had always intended my first book, *Broadmoor Revealed*, to be the starting point in a longer journey around Britain's Victorian asylums. However, it was written as a tour of some interesting cases rather than as the history of a subject, and of necessity it sketched over the mental health landscape in which Broadmoor was created. I meant to return to that landscape and provide a fuller description of it, and I wanted to do so with reference not only to Broadmoor but also to a community mental health hospital.

Life in the Victorian Asylum fulfils that aim; it defines the intricate worlds of Broadmoor and the other public asylums constructed in Britain during the nineteenth century. It unravels the knots of Victorian thinking about mental health care, explaining what asylum life was meant to achieve for patients. It does so in two parts. The first of these is an imitation of a modern treatment guide, such as might be written by a patient liaison service today for prospective clients. I have called that part a 'patient's handbook', and it adopts a Victorian tone and perspective, but it also acknowledges the new patient as a human being and attempts to address the sort of queries and concerns someone might have on entering an asylum.

The second part of *Life in the Victorian Asylum* is a discussion of the patient experience in the mid to late nineteenth century, as seen through early twenty-first century eyes. It includes a real-life history of Berkshire's own public asylum – Moulsford – and a note about how Broadmoor, the nation's criminal asylum, differed from other institutions. There is also a discussion about how time has weathered the beliefs and wisdoms of the Victorian age. Finally, it examines the legacy that Victorian health care has left behind it, and how the memories of the asylum are kept alive today.

Inevitably, a detailed description of asylum life should have a high human content. As permanent as the fixtures and fittings that adorned the wards, a constant stream of patients and staff flowed through the long corridors and occupied the chairs and benches in the day-rooms and airing courts. I hope that this book is more than just a physical description of a building and a routine, and that within each chapter you can sense the ghosts of those people for whom the asylum became at first a domicile and then a final resting place.

So many thousands of men, women and children passed through the doors of Victorian asylums and spent the rest of their lives removed from friends and family. It was an existence based on the idea of sanctuary within a refuge which, for many, became a terminus.

This book is for all those patients who never made it home.

Mark Stevens
Reading, January 2014

Part I

The Victorian Asylum Patient's Handbook

Dear New Patient,

Welcome to the Victorian asylum. We trust that your stay with us will be an improving one. We recognise that going into hospital can be a troubling experience, both for you and for your friends or family. It is our job to make this experience a calming and beneficial one. We want to assure you that we, the asylum staff, will dedicate ourselves to your well-being. We shall try to make you feel as comfortable as possible, while we endeavour to attend to all your medical needs.

As a first step, this book will help you to make sense of your new surroundings. It is designed to act as a manual, answering questions you may have about your treatment, care and opportunities and describing the buildings, facilities and staff. In short, we hope to prepare you for life inside the dormitories and wards in which our patients find themselves at rest.

With best regards for your healthy recovery,

Yours ever,

The Medical Superintendent

The Aims of the Asylum

We do not have an asylum mission statement, or a set of values embroidered on our letterheads. However, we do have some unspoken aims:

I.   To aid the recovery of the curable, helping them to live free both from mental illness and from treatment for it.
II. To create the best circumstances possible to help patients achieve recovery.
III. To recognise that some patients will remain incurable, and in such cases to continue to provide care, accommodation and support which allows them to be as comfortable as their condition permits.
IV. To ensure that if a patient is discharged, that they are not at risk of returning to the asylum.
V.   To prevent each patient's friends or family from being burdened with the care of the patient.

Every action that the asylum staff take is designed to help achieve these aims. In keeping with the trust in professional men so prevalent in this period, our staff believe implicitly that they know best and that their judgement ought never to be questioned.

The Popular Image of the Victorian Asylum

It may be that your family or friends have recounted what they believe you should expect on entering the asylum. They may have described it as the 'madhouse' or full of 'lunatics'; they may even have whispered tales of cruelty that made you anxious as your time here approached. Or it may be that you have read stories in the popular press about what life is like inside an asylum; stories which are not designed to set you at your ease, but which spread fear of the mentally ill and the conditions they are housed in. If this is so, then please do not be alarmed. Society finds it hard to understand your illness, and the result is that many stories of insanity are sensationalist in nature. They have been exaggerated to inspire the thrill of gossip or created with the aim of selling newspapers, and they do not convey an accurate picture.

The stories that you have heard almost certainly bear no relation to the realities of modern, Victorian health care. For example, you may have heard stories about lunatic patients being chained, left naked in their own filth, or paraded before a paying audience as a spectacle. Yet these practices belong to a different, more barbaric age. Since the early years of this century, physicians have treated those afflicted by the moon in a humane way, and for many years now restraint of any kind has been looked on as a defeat by men of science.

This is not London's infamous Bedlam, and you are not part of any circus freak show; instead, you are among a number of ordinary men and women who are no different from any other member of Victorian society. What sets you apart is only the disease from which you suffer and its chronic or acute symptoms. Your case need not be hopeless, and when the asylum doors close behind you they do not necessarily close forever.

In consequence, the asylum staff have a duty not to ridicule or imprison you but to help you to recover. Endeavour to keep this thought uppermost while your own mind is confused. Of course, there will be elements of both observation and security to any patient's stay, as these are a natural part of any asylum system, but such things are merely a necessary part of your treatment. Society has recognised that it may be more beneficial for you to reside in a hospital like this, both for your own protection and that of the wider community, so a degree of isolation is inevitable. Nevertheless, we will balance the effect of what may be seen as banishment with both positive interventions and opportunity.

A True Picture of the Asylum

Look around: you will see attractive, light and spacious rooms, rather different to the basic, dark and cramped accommodation in the workhouse, that other notable Victorian institution. The buildings here are pleasant; in the asylum, the patient is surrounded by the latest designs in nineteenth century architecture. Decorative, multi-coloured brickwork of sturdy and reliable construction forms the outer walls and draws the eye upwards.

The interiors are painted regularly, and augmented with ornate woodwork doorways, panels and skirtings, as well as comforting hearths to soothe and inspire the spirit. Large, multi-paned windows and high ceilings allow better circulation of the air and aid the eradication of disease. The latest in gas lighting provides relief from the dark, and warm air fans up from the floors through the use of patented boilers and cast iron grates.

Walk around the estate. Here, the grounds extend for acre upon acre, stretching so far that the boundaries are invisible. Close by the buildings are the enclosed airing courts, with winding paths and flower borders, and beyond them is leisure ground, lush, green and stocked with native trees and plants. You will have ready access to both these areas. If you enjoy outdoor work, then you may spend time also in our plots and fields, which lie barren in winter but burst with life in summer.

Take a deep breath of the pure, rural air. There are no factories here, no industrial smoke or foul smells to fog your brain and cause confusion, only the sweet whiff of rehabilitation emanates from the soil. You are the richest man, surrounded by the wealth of nature, in a place which invests only in good health.

The asylum is also a safe place. To grant asylum is to give protection and security, to offer a refuge from whatever threatens you, and once you are here we will watch over you and offer that refuge. The site is amply monitored by staff, who will continuously check that you are not at risk of harm, whether from yourself or others. We will not allow you to place yourself in any situation that could possibly be detrimental. We will also make sure there is no need for you to leave the premises, and that your freedom from the outside world is absolute.

This attention to your security extends to outside influence. Whilst we recognise that your family and friends will be concerned about your welfare, we cannot permit them to hamper your recovery. Any external correspondence or visitors will be carefully checked before contact is allowed. We are your physical and moral guardians, and we will not waver in our responsibility.

What we offer in return for your co-operation is the very latest in lunatic healthcare. Here you will have access to all the activities you need to improve your mental state. There are many different opportunities for industry and labour, so that whatever skills you have, we can find something to occupy you. There are also stimulating recreational activities, from parlour games to team sports and dramatics, and if these pursuits seem too strenuous, then a gentle walk around the grounds or a little friendly conversation can always be had to pass the hours in a productive manner.

There is far more going on here than you could possibly have imagined. You will also find that you are not alone but joining hundreds of fellow patients all affected by similar conditions, and all treated just the same. The male and female quarters are, of course, strictly separated, but otherwise there are many chances to enjoy social time and to bond with other members of your social class or degree of education. In many respects you will find our community no different to the one that you have left.

All that remains now is for you to join us and experience a daily life punctuated only by what will make you well.

You may find it so comforting that you never leave.

Chapter 1

Lunacy and Lunatics in Victorian England

You will be pleased to hear that it is a favourable time to be diagnosed as insane. Legislation has been passed to protect the lunatic, a great deal of public money is being invested in his care and also in research to improve treatment of conditions affecting the mind. Society has also become more aware and more tolerant of the range of mental illnesses recognised by modern science.

The nineteenth century has seen an enormous change in public perception of those who have lost their will or judgement. It is over a hundred years since the great men of the Enlightenment challenged us to employ reason in our quest for knowledge, and that idea is now at the heart of all we do. Gradually, reason has freed mankind from its bonds. The new, rational approach to your diagnosis and treatment has been influenced by wisdom and science rather than faith and superstition. We no longer believe that your soul is afflicted and understand that your illness is within your flesh and blood.

Sadly, much unnecessary suffering took place before the care of the insane caught up with the age of reason. Even in the early 1800s, many patients were left to fend for themselves in British cities, towns and villages. While the better-off could afford private care or family support, for most homes the burden of a lunatic child or spouse - requiring constant supervision and unable to contribute to the family income - caused great privation. Those patients lacking relatives or friends able to support them depended solely on charitable relief. A lifetime on the streets beckoned, though, because of their propensity for irrational action, lunatics also ended up confined in prisons. These were wretched places in which to shelter confused persons: generally dark, dirty and overcrowded, any form of treatment was impossible and many cries for help went unheard.

This is not to say that institutional care necessarily generated a better outcome than the gaol. Inside the few private asylums of the Georgian period, the outlook for a lunatic was often dramatically worse than for those subsisting outside, with custody and neglect the sole routine provided by physicians seeking financial bounty. Only a desperate case indeed would surrender itself for admission.

One unfortunate young pauper woman, Hannah Mills, was taken to the York County Asylum in 1790. She had been widowed and was suffering from an acute case of melancholy. Within weeks, Hannah was dead, the victim of a callous regime which spared all expense in managing its charges. Patients at York were dirty, malnourished and kept under restraint in an exercise of containment rather than care. Visitors were banned, and no physicians would attend the patients unless contracted by the governors; an untrained rogue was the patients' keeper. Profit had been put before people and with devastating effect. Public outrage ensued when Hannah's friends discovered the truth of the conditions that had caused her death. How could such abuse be permissible in prosperous eighteenth century England?

The remedy arrived by applying the new science of reason. Hannah Mills was a Quaker, and it was clear to all her friends that those who ran the York Asylum had not followed any basic teachings from that religion. For Quakers believe that God is in all of us, even those who have become insane. It follows that the lunatic is no different from the rest of men, and that they should be treated like any other neighbour. This starting point for rational thought heralded in an entirely new system of care. By 1796, Hannah's fellow Quaker William Tuke had opened a new asylum in York. The Retreat would be completely different from any English asylum that had gone before it.

Within twenty years, The Retreat had transformed the management of those who were mentally ill and the way that they were perceived. Rather than condemn the lunatic like an unreformed prisoner, William Tuke's regime sought to treat him as an innocent, and to boost the morale of all those who crossed its threshold by providing a uniform kindness. Tuke's 'moral treatment' offered the hope of a cure and the certainty of compassion, and, above all, it reduced the stigma of insanity.

Of course, it took some time for these new ideas to become widely accepted. The authorities running Bethlem, London's oldest asylum (known also as Bedlam), were found guilty in 1815 of much the same practices as the York County Asylum had been in 1790. One patient, William Norris, was discovered by inspectors unable to move, his arms fastened to his sides and his neck chained to an iron bar. Norris' treatment met with widespread condemnation, and slowly the medical establishment adopted Tuke's reforms. Finally, in 1839, John Conolly, physician in charge at the Hanwell Asylum, tore up all his attendants' mechanisms of restraint. His action was a symbolic declaration that all the country's lunatics should be free.

Today, the scandals of the past have been left behind; neglect, mistreatment and bondage are gone; in their place we offer attention, treatment and refuge.

How Public Asylums Came into Being

For centuries, the care of lunatics was of no interest to the state. Such provision as there was came about through the auspices of private charities or private speculators. It is well-known that any alienist, or mind-doctor, was obliged to turn a surplus if he wished to continue in his business, and if that surplus did not come about through benefaction, then it had to be encouraged through careful management. There was no incentive to cure; indeed, the reverse was often of greater pecuniary value.

It is easy to see in retrospect that an unregulated system of care is no system at all; to engineer abuse one may just as well let any profession moderate itself. Abuse certainly followed, reported in cases such as that of Mrs Hawsley, a woman tricked into confinement in a Chelsea madhouse for no other reason than that her mother considered her a drunk. There, she discovered that a fellow inmate, Mrs Smith, displayed no obvious symptoms of madness. The latter woman had been incarcerated solely because her husband wished to be rid of her and could afford to pay the requisite fee.

The discovery of many similar cases led eventually to statute. The Madhouses Act of 1774 began a system of licensing and inspection for the various private asylums operating throughout the country. Bad practice, such as admitting sane people who were merely inconvenient to their families, or treating patients inhumanely could result in the refusal of a licence. For the first time, British lunatics had someone to watch over them.

This was just as well, for the turn of the century led to a dramatic rise in patient numbers. One key event raised the public consciousness of the mad within society: the assault by James Hadfield on King George III. Hadfield, a young soldier who fired two pistols at His Majesty in May 1800, was unusual in that he ended up in Bethlem. It must be said, with great regret, that at this time a far larger number of the insane were placed within parish workhouses and county gaols. This was an expensive and ultimately fruitless outcome, as no lunatics were being cured by custody.

A select committee of the House of Commons was created to suggest a solution to this problem, and in 1808, all the counties of England and Wales were empowered to build public asylums. Few chose to do so. Many of the county justices were not convinced that money spent on asylums was money well spent. The counterargument, of course, is that their residents will inevitably find themselves inside one institution or another, and that respite care in an asylum is no more expensive than providing extra beds in a workhouse or prison, though with the greater possibility of a beneficial outcome. In the end, not spending money on public asylums became a false economy.

When Nottinghamshire opened a building for sixty patients in 1811, it became the first county to pay for the upkeep of some of its lunatics through the parish poor rates. It is easy to forget just how recent this development was, but it has since become the standard model. Local taxation now pays for virtually all the patients in our mental health accommodation. The professional management of relief brought about through the poor law also made reliance on untrained volunteers a thing of the past. The future would be one of skilled public service.

Nevertheless, it took time for universal care to be established and, unfortunately, fear was once again the spark. There was the case of Edward Oxford, the young boy who shot, attempting to gain notoriety, at our pregnant Queen in 1840; or Daniel McNaughten, the Scottish wood-turner who, convinced that he was persecuted by the government, killed the secretary of Sir Robert Peel in 1843. The actions of these two men, though at odds with the harmlessness of the vast majority of lunatics, were actions for which society demanded a response. Parliamentary inquiry was inevitable, and brought with it an insistence that every county or named borough should provide an asylum for its populace or establish a contract to house its lunatics with a neighbouring authority.

The result was the framework that we have in place today, based on the two great statutes of Victorian health care: the Lunatic Asylums Act of 1845 and its companion, the Lunacy Act.

The Present Statutory Framework on Lunacy

Like every patient, your position has its roots in the Lunacy Act. This piece of legislation governs everything, from the means by which you came here to those by which you may leave; all the paperwork that controls your comings and going is contained within it.

The Act also delegates many powers to the Commissioners in Lunacy, and they produce rules establishing precisely how we should build public asylums, how we should care for patients, how we should manage our affairs and how we should report our findings. From their offices in Whitehall, these highly-qualified legal and medical men exercise a tight control over the treatment of lunatics across the country. If you stay here any length of time, you may meet some of the Commissioners during one of their annual inspections.

At a more local level, our own committee of visitors is also empowered to operate under the Act. These men are all appointed by the local justices and it is to them that the superintendent directly reports. They are men of property and status, used to committee work and to devoting themselves to public service. They are ideally placed to look after your interests while you are here. As their name suggests, the committee members are also regular visitors to the asylum, and you may see the superintendent escorting one or two of their number from time to time.

The asylum that you are now in was established as a result of the 1845 Lunatic Asylums Act. This statute was designed to end the system by which a patient's chance of treatment rested unfairly on the accident of where he or she lived. The Act finally created a national system of care for pauper lunatics (those relieved by expenditure from the rates) based on a uniform model. Henceforth, sufficient accommodation was to be provided by every county or city throughout the land – and asylums were soon everywhere.

Before the introduction of the Asylums Act, only around 5,000 lunatic patients were cared for in publicly-funded asylum beds, in contrast with the 12,000 or so lunatics who could be counted among the inmates of the country's workhouses and gaol. Many patients suffering insanity or imbecility were being denied proper care, and the most satisfactory way of providing places for them was by creating entirely new buildings. Because most workhouses did not have sufficient room on site for the additional space required, and the few existing public asylums were not placed equidistantly around the country, fresh establishments were used to bridge the gap. The result was an enormous undertaking of public works.

Since 1845 some sixty new asylums have been built across England and Wales. These state-of-the-art facilities came to be provided more and more locally, so that patients do not have to travel miles from home to receive treatment and their friends and family are able to visit. These new institutions are usually placed in pleasant, rural surroundings – 'fixed upon an airy and healthy situation', to quote the original 1808 Act – and have rapidly become a fixture in Victorian society.

You may be surprised to discover how much financial support the public purse provides to fund your treatment. The generous expenditure upon the lunatic is in contrast to the general parsimony of the poor law and the workhouse system. Some three times the weekly allowance for a pauper in the workhouse will be spent on you, in recognition that you are not responsible for the condition in which you find yourself. Your economic failings are innocent; you are the deserving poor. It would be a grave error to weaken you further when instead we might improve your health and return you to the workforce, ready to make a contribution to society once more.

The result of this approach is that the pauper patient in our charge is somewhat different from the pauper of the workhouse. Many respectable working men and women become our patients; these are not people who have fallen slowly on hard times but individuals who have suddenly become ill. Insanity is something that compels the conscientious labourer or artisan as much as the shiftless vagabond or thief. If your family is unable to pay for the care you need, or you have not the means, then the ratepayers will intercede on your behalf. It is not our purpose to exclude sufferers, rather, our job is to cater for all.

You may have previously read about the growth in asylum care during recent decades and marvelled at it. At the present rate of increase we shall have around 100,000 patients within asylums nationally by the turn of the twentieth century. That is a large number, and to anticipate it new asylums are built to house anywhere between 700 and 1,000 residents beneath their roofs. It is a significant change from the more modest intention of 1845 to find an extra 12,000 beds across the country.

Although the scale of mental health treatment was previously unimagined by our forebears, it must be seen in context. Great men have argued convincingly that an evil can exist for many years without our knowledge of it, and insanity is one such evil, left unexplored and unexplained for far too long. Only now are we beginning to understand the full range of connected illnesses and so it is inevitable that diagnoses should increase. When compared to our total population, it is true that, proportionately, the incidence of lunacy has increased slightly, but even now, in the latter half of the nineteenth century, the number of lunatics contained within asylums accounts for only one in every 400 of Her Majesty's subjects.

Chapter 2

Admission

You have been admitted to the asylum because someone was worried about you. It is likely that you have exhibited behaviour that caused anxiety or alarm to those closest to you. Perhaps you have been very melancholy lately, or very excited; perhaps you have acted in a way that is unbecoming to a man or woman; perhaps you threatened someone with violence, or even hurt them; perhaps you have endured terrors, fearing that your food is poisoned, that you are being followed or otherwise persecuted. You may have said that you wished to undertake some grand scheme, deliver a message to an important personage or foil some conspiracy you have discovered.

This behaviour may have come about after some traumatic event, such as a bereavement, shock or disappointment in love, but equally it may have emerged through no discernible factor. Of course, there may be another precursor to your admission: you may have been apprehended by the police, found wandering as a tramp or vagrant or even sent to gaol and found unfit to be released into society.

Your behaviour may well have been observed for some time before any action was taken. Initially, your family and friends might have made suggestions for the improvement of your health and, if they were able to afford it, called a doctor to attend you. He would have offered practical advice such as a period of rest or a change of scenery, or suggested that you abstain from alcohol or religious activities, or avoid potentially upsetting situations.

Almost inevitably, these interventions failed. Yet, if those for whom you care most have been unable to obtain respite for you, then they must not be blamed. The workings of the mind do not easily allow a non-professional interpretation. However desirous your family may have been of keeping you at home, when it became harder for them to do so their thoughts turned naturally to possible alternatives.

Involving the Poor Law Officers

The decision to ask for assistance was not taken lightly. Your family only took action once they reluctantly concluded that domestic care was no longer practicable. Perhaps they found it difficult to provide food or board for you, especially after the loss of your wages. They might also have struggled to find the time or safe environment required to offer care. It is possible too that they recognised your domestic surroundings were only likely to nurture your illness, rather than resolve it.

At some point your behaviour was perceived as creating a burden. Having made this decision, your relatives or friends were obliged to speak to the relieving officer of the local poor law union to ask for help.

The relieving officer makes recommendations as to whom shall receive relief from the union, and what form that relief should take, as well as assessing those persons who wish to enter the workhouse. He recognises that the public purse does not open for everyone who needs assistance, and that each case must be scrupulously examined. The relieving officer works closely with his chaplain and the workhouse medical officer when considering the matter of asylum care. That triumvirate of authority holds much power over the allocation of help for lunatics. Unless your family was able to afford a doctor, then the relieving officer ensures that for the first time you had the benefit of a learned, medical opinion on your case.

Now that the doctors' profession is regulated by the Medical Act of 1858, any union medical officer will be perfectly able to reflect on the symptoms of your case. Though it is unlikely that he attended a medical school, he will doubtless have served a thorough apprenticeship with an experienced physician and learned his trade on the job. Indeed, as he is almost certainly a private practitioner contracted to his local union, the medical officer will, most likely, have experience of lunatics as part of his commercial work.

The medical officer is instructed by the relieving officer to visit any prospective asylum patients for a thorough examination. If the patient is a workhouse inmate, then the examination is held within that institution. If visiting a lunatic patient at home, the medical officer anticipates the need to undertake the consultation in a domestic setting, within the living room or kitchen. They are not influenced by your class or status; by the appearance of your clothes or shoes or by the contents of your larder.

Since the middle of the century, doctors attending lunatics have been asked to make direct observations of the patient's symptoms, and usually base their opinion on the record of these observations. Observations that tend towards a diagnosis of insanity include, though are not limited to:

Incessant chatter and the use of inappropriate or over-familiar language, laughing or singing without obvious cause or motive.

A loss of strength or will, resulting in a failure to be active in chores or employment or to interact with those around you.

A belief that fraudulent enemies unknown are depriving you of something that is rightfully yours, or are trying to poison or otherwise attack you. Typically, a patient in this condition may have made threats to harm someone they know or to destroy their property, believing them to be part of the conspiracy against them.

Being found wandering without seeming to have an aim or direction, and usually in a state of inadequate dress.

A fear or dread of something being about to befall you, no matter how unlikely, such as your bed catching fire or being infected by some fanciful disease.

Holding some unusual desires or notions, such as the need to act as a messenger or a belief that you can predict high tides.

Unusual facial expressions, such as constant grimacing, twitching or other violent movements or the acting out of imaginary fancies.

If a parent, especially a mother, ceasing to show interest in the care of your children. In extreme cases, you may have threatened or attempted to harm your child.

Although hearsay is no longer considered sufficient evidence of insanity, physicians would be remiss if they did not also ask your family or friends for their own observations to build a picture of your state of mind. A basic family history is taken to ascertain whether insanity has been found elsewhere within your family. The doctors also enquire whether you are epileptic, dangerous or of intemperate habits.

The answers to these questions help to inform your prognosis, and without prejudice, the medical officer will reach a conclusion on your situation. If he believes that he has observed evidence of insanity, then within the week you will be examined by another doctor from a different practice. If both physicians agree that you have become insane, the relieving officer must assess your eligibility for asylum treatment. He has already ascertained your legal place of settlement – that is, the place on which the financial burden of your relief will fall – to make sure that your relief is his responsibility, rather than that of another union. Should the latter be the case, efforts are made to speedily effect your removal to that place. The relieving officer works quickly, as there is a penalty placed upon him should he dally and, in theory, the law allows him only three days to arrange for all his enquiries.

Relieving officers are well-known to prefer cheaper workhouse care to prevail for local people suffering from afflictions of the mind, if they can reasonably allow it. Theirs is not a medical profession, but rather that of regulator of the poor. Somewhat bleaker, and with no grounds around it, patients within the workhouse infirmary find care provided only by recruits from amongst the able poor. Rarely are paid nurses employed within a workhouse, and there is often only one doctor to cater for the whole establishment. Patients are surrounded by physical maladies, the aged, the infirm and the disabled. The dormitories are damp and overcrowded. The diet is spare and the day intended solely for monotonous, unrewarding labour such as cleaning, breaking stones or picking oakum.

The workhouse is no bastion of health; it is not a place of cure, but a wretched stable for those who lack a roof. Nevertheless, it is a regrettable fact that even today, many of the indigent and destitute within the workhouse population are also sufferers of insanity. We must constantly urge the relieving officers that if treatment of a lunatic is required, then it must be given in its proper setting: an asylum.

It is not for the relieving officers or the medical men to sanction your admission here; rather, they must defer to the magistrates. The 1845 Lunacy Act requires that a justice of the peace receives the physicians' certificates and makes an order to admit you to an asylum. This safeguard ensures that only by due process of law are you authorised to be removed from society. It is not necessary for the magistrate to question you or those applying for your admission. Instead, he simply checks that the paperwork was correctly completed before signing the order laid before him, and then the relieving officer is instructed to arrange for your admission here.

At no stage of this process does a patient have any contact with the medical officers in this asylum. That is quite proper, as we wish to place ourselves entirely outside the process of admission. It is our job to manage your condition rather than to seek your custody; to treat, but not to seek out patients who require treatment. We place our confidence in our poor law colleagues to make the right decisions on our behalf.

Arriving at the Asylum

The relieving officer arranges your transport and accompanies you on the journey. Female patients are additionally accompanied by one of the workhouse's female volunteers. Your care is their responsibility until you are handed over to us. Together with your attendants, patients may journey by horse-drawn carriage, by rail, or a combination of the two. Our own horse-drawn carriage seats four and is open or closed depending on the season, but always affords a good view of the local countryside. Travelling by carriage is generally considered to be a healthy experience, providing opportunity for fresh air, and regular stops for sustenance or rest en route.

Most union towns also have railway stations, offering the opportunity of travelling to the asylum more swiftly by locomotive. The railway is an assault upon the senses, and the fumes of the engine and the noise of the pistons can be quite traumatic when newly experienced. The station itself is unlikely to be grand, but even so paupers must wait while the first and second class ticket passengers board, before they are allowed out onto the platform and into the third class coach.

The workhouse staff will place you on a wooden bench, wedged securely between them. As the coach shudders and jolts, you may feel as though you are being pulled at an unnatural speed. Hopefully, the oblivious expressions of those around you provide some comfort, and the enclosed wagon spares you from catching sight of the scenery rushing past and noticing the sensation of hurry.

By whatever means you travel here, a luggage allowance is made available. Of necessity it is limited, though perhaps your sole personal possessions are either worn on your frame or can be contained within a small parcel. You will also notice that at least one member of staff from the workhouse brought their own bag; they are obliged to oversee your admission and, as a result, will need to spend the night here.

As you approach the asylum, you may strain to look out of the carriage window. Your first sight is of the gatehouse, a small, domestic building, much like any other brick and tile house, with a sloping roof and sash windows. Its only notable feature is a first-floor room looking onto the road by which you arrived, as well as the driveway leading to the asylum itself. This is where the gatekeeper lives and performs his duty to watch those who come and go. All carriages stop here before entering, and the union officer speaks to the gatekeeper for permission to move through.

When the driver turns the carriage through the gates the asylum buildings open up before you. As the horse trots, crunching on the gravel drive while the wheels turn rhythmically behind him, the eye is drawn to the three-storey structure stretching out in front. In many ways, an asylum is designed to look a little like a country house; of course, it is large and imposing, but it should also be welcoming and uplifting, with a sense of grandeur. The architecture is more decorative than that of the workhouse, the windows larger and more airy. Though you may not notice it initially, the materials too are of a high quality. External doors are oak, and stone augments the brickwork; the multiple chimney breasts suggest a constant source of heat within.

By now, your carriage has stopped beside the entrance and the door of the trap is unlocked for you. Alongside your companions, you are escorted down its steps and across the gravel to the entrance door. As you take your first step inside the wood-panelled hallway you may notice some of the asylum staff moving back and forth, engaged in their labours. No one will remark upon your appearance, and all will remain calm as you are invited to take a seat in the waiting room.

The Formalities of Admission

You may be feeling disorientated by the time you arrive and, realising this, we attempt to make the admissions process as simple as possible. Your arrival should be expected – though, occasionally, relieving officers have been known to spring surprise admissions upon us, an action for which they will be censured – and your reception is noted. The union officials are greeted by one of the asylum staff and the paperwork that accompanied you is taken off to our clerk's office, where it forms the first part of your patient record.

Here is a typical admissions form:

Name of patient:
Sex and Age:
Married, widowed or single:
Condition of life, and previous occupation (if any):
Religious persuasion:
Previous place of abode:
Whether first attack:
Age (if known) of first attack:
Duration of existing attack:
Supposed cause:
Whether subject to epilepsy:
Whether suicidal:
Whether dangerous to others:
Parish or Union to which the lunatic is chargeable:

Your companions will either leave the asylum now or be taken off to our guest accommodation, while you are invited into the 'receiving room', which is situated close to the offices of our medical men. On the walls you can see cabinets containing bottles and boxes, as well as shelves of books, some comprising hand-written records, and a table and a chair. The assistant medical officer will be present and also, if you are a female patient, either the housekeeper or another member of the female staff.

In the receiving room you are asked to stand on a special machine that combines scales with a slide rule to record your weight and measure your height. Next to the receiving room is a bathroom, and here you are invited to disrobe and bathe. We also make a note of any distinguishing marks or features you possess and look for evidence of lice, or known contagious diseases such as scarlet fever, measles, diphtheria, erysipelas, typhoid fever or chickenpox.

If you are suffering from any of these afflictions, then you present a danger of infection to the other patients, and your first days here will be spent quarantined in the infirmary ward. In this case it will not be possible to retain your clothes for future use; instead, they will be burnt in the boiler house. Similarly, it may be necessary to take shears to your hair to assist with the treatment of any infestation, though in most cases effective remedies can be administered without such extreme action.

After your bath you will be given a set of asylum clothing to wear. Your old clothes, if they are clean, and possessions will be taken away to the asylum stores, where they will await your departure at a future date. If it is safe for you to retain any of your possessions, then they will be made available to you in due course. Meanwhile, you will be taken off to the admissions ward.

This is the point at which you leave your previous life behind and take the first step towards convalescence and recovery. You have become an asylum patient and you are now in our care.

Chapter 3

Accommodation

One of the first things you notice on entering the asylum is the scale of our enterprise. Far larger than a union workhouse, dispensary or charitable hospital, this institution more closely resembles a great estate, with a country house and satellite outbuildings. In truth, this is an almost inevitable consequence of the Commissioners' rules governing the arrangement and construction of our buildings. Wise men have detailed exactly what constituent elements make an asylum work, and these instructions were passed on to our own architects and surveyors as they laid out our property. Some explanation of their thinking may assist you to comprehend the substance of your new home.

Our site

It is a recognised principle that asylums should be built only on land possessing natural qualities which afford the greatest opportunities for recovery and convalescence. The first Asylums Act of 1808 stipulated this, and modern guidance has been offered as to what might constitute a suitable site.

Of course, no asylum should be built close to anything that might be considered a nuisance, and nuisances can manifest themselves in many ways. The great inventions of the industrial world have brought with them as by-products the fiercest noises and the foulest smells. Therefore, industrial devices are not welcome beside our own endeavours – no factories, mines or steam machinery will be found adjacent to our borders; no offensive discharges are welcome in our air or water. Neither will you find an asylum built on low ground and overlooked, or local persons allowed a right of way across our roads or paths. Tranquillity is a great prescription for the unquiet mind and its dose should not be compromised.

Often, you will find an asylum built on chalk or rocky ground, and placed upon an eminence. The reasons for this are partly practical. While the command of an inspiring view, preferably to the south, is of benefit to the spirit, it also affords the necessary drop to take advantage of gravity's assistance with the inevitable waste flow from our sewage pipes. Water ingress and egress are important factors.

To date, we have dug a total of three wells on our site to ensure an adequate supply of clean water for washing or drinking. The first well was sunk to the depth of some 40 feet, which yields a maximum of nearly 2,000 gallons an hour. This well is replenished every autumn, while the two additional wells are used only in the driest summers. The water is pumped from these wells into two great cisterns, one within our north tower, the other in the south. Smaller hot water cisterns in each tower are heated by the boilers. In the event of extreme weather, we also have access to an underground rainwater tank, filled from the gutters and downpipes on the building roofs.

We have no lofty grounds as such, but our buildings are situated on the elevated portion of our site, set some 400 feet back from the public highway that passes by our entrance gates, and from which we are divided by a wire fence. What we lack in altitude we make up for with a private estate of 80 acres, sloping down towards the water meadows a short distance from one of England's greatest rivers. Generally, water features are to be avoided in asylums on the grounds of safety; here, however, we are obliged to work with nature, and the flow of the river offers up a wondrous sight, whilst remaining at a safe distance from our gardens.

The view across the south side of the estate rises up across the river to rolling folds of the greenest hills, which are cloaked in natural forest. You can watch the sun rise behind these undulations in the morning until it passes before them in the afternoon, casting long shadows of grey and pink across the straightest spears of the stateliest trees. A handsome iron viaduct crosses the river to the south-east, and distant billows of smoke rise rhythmically from passing engines.

We are also on prime agricultural land, which is of great importance for producing asylum food. The whole of the acreage extends roughly half a mile from north to south and one quarter mile from east to west. As very little of this space is built upon, oats, wheat and barley are cultivated above ground for use in bulking out the asylum diet, while potatoes are grown beneath.

Our position is additionally prudent in terms of transportation. Though removed from the nearest centres of population, we remain within a mile of a mainline railway station, and the rails skirt the edge of our estate. A stout iron fence prevents ready access to the railway embankment, however. The main road nearby also brings much traffic from the closest town, some two miles distant, and so your friends and family will find it easy to travel here.

The grounds are divided into sections with different uses. On either side of the asylum driveway are landscaped areas dedicated to grass and native trees both deciduous and evergreen. These not only shield the buildings from the road, but provide a canopy of grandeur on the north side without depriving us of light. The drive is of gravel, laid on earth, so that heavy rainfall should not prevent the path from being usable. Similar precautions have been taken on the private walkways around the grounds.

Immediately to the south-east of our main building is a formal garden, where pathways, lawns and beds provide some seasonal colour. Convalescing patients will find vantage points on the seats and benches to enjoy the fresh air. Trees have also been planted to shade the glare of the sun. Enclosed between the gardens and the accommodation blocks are four walled airing courts, two for the men and two for the women, which consist of more simple spaces, bounded by walls and planted with shrubs. Some of these courts allow the convalescent patients to shelter, while others give the more troublesome cases a safer means of enjoying the great outdoors.

You will notice also the kitchen gardens, stretching on either side of the pathway that leads down from the main block towards the river. Though the river is most strictly out of bounds to patients, within the kitchen gardens patient labour is encouraged. Amongst fruit trees and bushes is a small orchard of cooking apples and the annual multitude of root and sprouting vegetables. These patches of soil lie barren in winter, but for the spring and summer months they are ablaze with colour and alive with insects.

The recommendation of the Commissioners in Lunacy states that an asylum site should provide a ratio of one acre of land for every four patients – an abundance of open space. The importance of our grounds cannot be stressed enough; they provide not just room for supplies, but, we hope, enough space for your mind to regain its former bearings.

The Asylum Buildings

Aside from the opulence of the principal block, our buildings are much like those you might see in any town or village. Let us deal first with the structures placed irregularly around the grounds. To one side of the entrance drive sits the courtyard, around which the farm buildings and the dairy are arranged. These are simple, single-storey structures, providing shelter to livestock. There is a covered stables too, for the asylum horses and those of visitors. Carriages are unharnessed in the courtyard and then stored beside the stables, while the dairy – the largest single part of the complex – provides accommodation for the cows and for their milking, with a pathway to the fields for grazing just beyond it.

A little further on is the asylum gasworks, which appear slightly out of proportion with the miniature farm, as their rounded, brick chimneys tower significantly higher than the other buildings. We create our gas by burning coal, and the coal gas is stored in large containers, the area of which is out of bounds for patients. Opposite the farm and gasworks, on the other side of the asylum drive, is the chapel, with a gravelled pathway leading towards it. The chapel's varicoloured brick walls are set against a deeply sloping roof of grey slate tiles, and the whitewashed roof beam ends extend to meet the slates like teeth protruding from an upper lip.

The chapel may be entered through the vast east door, and inside, you can appreciate the coloured light that radiates from the stained glass windows, which are shaped in gothic arches. At the altar end, patterns emerge where the sun leaks in through the etched glass. Above you is a vaulted ceiling, with oak rafters sitting on corbels of Portland stone, while at ground level are bench pews fashioned from elm. We are obliged to provide seating in the chapel for three quarters of our patient number, over 200 men and women. The staff sit at the front, perpendicular to the patients and able to observe them. Opposite the pulpit is a wooden harmonium, while to the side hangs a notice board, the numbers of the hymns from the recent service slotted into the grooves within it.

On leaving the chapel, we may take the pathway back towards the main drive and the asylum entrance. As we return, it is worth remarking on two areas that are slightly distinct from the principal accommodation: the engine house and workshops for the male patients, and the asylum laundry. We come to the laundry first, as it is nearest to the chapel. An efficient asylum laundry is of great importance, and foul linen should be quickly cleansed.

There are various rooms within the laundry; some have wooden washing troughs, supplied with hot and cold taps, in which linen is washed with soap and then rinsed. The air is moist and humid here, even with the windows open. We find that it is generally more agreeable for our laundresses to undertake washing by hand, although we have recently installed two of Haden's revolving machines, which allow for a greater volume of items in one wash. At first, we found that steam from these machines caused condensation on the copper pipes running above the drums. This condensation dripped upon the laundry maids and the garments, staining the latter with an iron hue and, as a result, it was necessary to move the pipework into adjacent rooms.

The room immediately beside the wash rooms is used for mangling with a centrifugal wringer, which is a more reliable aid to drying than a hand mangle. To one side of the room are two drying closets into which steam is delivered, with an outdoor yard nearby for drying in the summer months, and a room for ironing linen.

To the other side of the asylum entrance is the engine house and workshops on the male side. The steam for the drying closets is provided by the engine here. Inside the single-storey building with a high, vaulted roof, coal is added each day to one of the boilers, which powers the great steam engine and its pumps. Thus heat is transferred to the cisterns and pipes in the living accommodation. The boilers are used alternately so that their working life might be extended; their room is ventilated by another vast chimney. The engine house operates at a tremendous temperature, while its noisy, thunderous occupant can roar like a dragon. Attached to it is a hooter that is used as the asylum alarm and sounded in emergency, to draw staff towards the main block.

Next to the boiler room is a store for the mountain of shiny black fuel ready to be consumed. Hundreds of tons of coal are delivered each year for burning in the boilers or the stoves of the main building. There are other coal stores around the site but this is the largest, and it is tended during the working day by a patient who helps the stoker.

In the other half of this house of industry lie the shops for shoemaking, painting, carpentry and upholstery, as well as a tailor's and a blacksmith's forge. Unlike the laundry, there is no mechanisation within these workshops and tools are provided for work by hand. Some half a dozen male patients may be found at any time in these shops, helping the artisan attendants that we employ.

The Principal Block

Now we have completed our tour of the out-buildings on the site, we will return to the main entrance. You will notice that our principal block is also constructed from brick, in the fashionable, gothic revivalist style. It resembles a fine house far more than an austere workhouse.

The Commissioners in Lunacy expound much advice about an asylum's principal accommodation, and we have followed this carefully. The block is constructed towards the northern end of the estate, leaving the expanse of uplifting grounds towards the south unimpeded. Then, in keeping with the use of southerly views to promote better health, our officers' administrative quarters have all been placed on the north side of the building beside the main door. Here is the wood-panelled committee room where our visitors meet; here also are the offices of those who are constantly engaged in the management of this institution – the medical superintendent and his assistant officer, the asylum steward, and the clerk. The superintendent's domestic accommodation is within a wing branching off this main entrance.

The structure allows for the seamless integration of work and home life for the staff. Within the walls are additional furnished living quarters for all the unmarried senior staff. Their rooms are commensurate with the status in life that these gentlemen (and lady) have achieved, and they are not at liberty to better the fittings without a reference to the committee of visitors, who will form a view of what might be acceptable.

The same approach to decoration is evident throughout the patient accommodation. Whilst we strive to provide an attractive, bright ambience at all times, we are obliged to give consideration to the limits of the public's generosity. Any object must have a clear use, any ornamentation justified likewise. That is not to suggest that our wards have an unfinished air, as skirtings, architraves and other woodwork are all provided in line with the best of domestic architectural practice. Similarly, doors and windows are of solid wood, though not adorned as you might expect within finer family homes.

The main asylum building consists of three storeys, with the second and third devoted chiefly to sleeping accommodation, while the entrance level is given over mostly to living space required throughout the daylight hours. The patients' accommodation within the asylum divides roughly into one-third for watched patients and two-thirds for those who can be allowed some degree of freedom. The watched encompass those who are sick, as well as those recently admitted or who must be prevented from causing injury to themselves or others. The patients in possession of greater freedom include those at labour, the more composed, or those who have recovered from their symptoms and are now convalescing.

Around the square core of the asylum ground floor runs a wide, enclosed corridor, illuminated at either end by a large window or glazed partition, and which forms a simple route around the centre of the building. In common with the rest of the asylum accommodation, it has a generous ceiling height of fifteen feet, allowing for circulation of air and a sense of space. The walls are plastered and whitewashed, while floorboards of seasoned oak have been laid. These are robust, pliant and also easy to clean without the application of water. Beneath them, air moves throughout the masonry and adds to the thorough ventilation of the building.

You will rarely see this central corridor unless you are brought through it for some purpose, perhaps to see the visitors, the superintendent or for a meeting. There are two reasons for this: first, the corridor provides access only to the offices, stores and staff rooms in the midst of the asylum and second, it is a neutral space between the great divide within the asylum, the separation of the male and female patients. For an axis can be run down the centre of this building that splits the accommodation belonging to the men from that of the women. This is a requisite and sensible precaution for control, as well as for the better protection of modesty. Yet it is also for your better health, as while men and women may enjoy each other's society, the accompanying complications can be detrimental to their mental wellbeing.

The only spaces to which patients on both sides of the corridor have recourse are the dining room and recreational hall. The dining room is designed to accommodate the entire asylum population, and each side has separate tables and benches for its own use. When we originally opened the asylum this room was cleared of furniture when entertainments were staged, but we now have the benefit of a discrete hall behind the dining room, connected with it by sliding doors. This hall has a stage and storage area for theatrical equipment, dressing rooms, and sufficient space for temporary seating.

The kitchen is accessible from the dining hall by serving hatches through which the food is passed. For ease of cleaning, the lower parts of the kitchen walls and its floor are tiled. Its working area has two substantial cooking ranges, each with a brick and iron oven and two boilers, heated by steam from the range. Vast quantities of vegetables are cooked on further boilers in the kitchen scullery, preventing the smell of cooking from overpowering the dining hall. There is a general store for groceries, and meat and dairy larders, with ventilation shafts to bring in air and keep produce cool.

The dining room and recreation hall are at the southerly end of the central corridor. Branching off to the east and west are two more divisions: covered walkways, leading off towards the south blocks and the north blocks of the asylum, where the patient accommodation is located.

The arrangement and contents of each block are broadly similar. Their names arise, as you might suppose, from their aspects. The south blocks have views over the asylum gardens and across the river, while the north block looks laterally towards the chapel, on the female side, and the farm on the male. In the larger south blocks convalescing and recently admitted patients reside, while the north blocks house those with more active and destructive forms of insanity.

Fanning out across the north and south blocks are the day-rooms for each sex, which also provide access to the grounds or the enclosed airing courts. The day-rooms afford no less than forty square feet for each patient and there is one for every ward, so that patients do not have to encounter those with different needs. These rooms are intended to help patients socialise during the day.

A wooden bead painted bright blue runs around the day-room walls at a height of five feet; above it the wall is whitewashed, below it is a warm, stone colour. The rooms have large, oak-framed windows, which open with a sash to afford liberal intake of fresh air. There are bay windows with seating built into them. All window openings on the ground floor are at a low level, so that the drop is not so great as to facilitate accidents. A fire stove is the centrepiece of each room. These stoves also heat the air drawn from outside the building and deliver it through grates placed around the day-room. The stoves are surrounded by an oak mantelpiece, and in all but wards for the most destructive patients, the mantelpiece is topped by a mirror framed in polished birch.

The rooms are lit by coal gas from our own works, which burns with great intensity to produce an excellent light; modern production methods have mostly removed the slightly sour, sulphurous smell with which it was long associated. Candles are on hand for use in case of an interrupted supply.

We strive overall for a look of domesticity and comeliness. In each day-room there is a variety of seating, with birch settees, high and low-backed chairs, and some padded smoking chairs beside sturdy tables. The latter may be decked with brightly-covered tablecloths, in colours that do not clash tempestuously with those of the room; while small card tables are supplied for writing or playing games. Some low chairs with padded backs and arms are available to more infirm patients.

As far as it is safe to do so, decorations to improve the atmosphere or articles for the amusements of patients will be placed within the day-rooms. The former include such items as potted plants or caged singing birds, while among the latter might be books or papers on an appropriate stand or case, or card or other games. Engravings of humorous or contemplative scenes have been hung in generous, attractive frames upon the walls. A letter box is provided, either in the room itself or the attendants' office, for patients' use.

Attached to each day-room is a small, tiled scullery equipped with a stove and sink. These sculleries are not accessible to patients, but allow the attendants to provide hot water throughout the day, or to prepare small amounts of food, if necessary. A serving hatch from each opens onto its adjacent day-room.

The windows of the day-rooms look out on to the airing courts. Each day-room also has a door that opens out on to the airing courts, and these doors may be unlocked all day on the less secure wards, or unlocked on the more secure wards when the attendants are ready for patients to take a turn outdoors. Access to all rooms on some wards is controlled via door locks; if you are placed on a restricted ward, you will need to be escorted either to or from your day-room by the staff.

The Upper Floors

Although some of our dormitories are at ground level, it is on the two upper floors that you will find the bulk of our sleeping accommodation. These are reached via one of a number of staircases at either end of the covered walkways. Each is enclosed within its own well, so that patients are never at risk of falling from a height, and a handrail is provided opposite the side where a banister might usually be found.

It is probably in one of the upstairs rooms that you will be allotted your own, regulated space. Overall, we may house a maximum of 285 patients at any time. There are slightly more rooms on the female side than the male, in keeping with the greater number of female patients expected within an asylum. By far the larger number of our beds are laid out within dormitories, and it is in one of these that you will spend most – if not all – your nights here. Dormitories of between eight and fifteen beds provide sleeping accommodation for 222 of our patients and, though space is shared, you are guaranteed a minimum of 600 square feet for your comfort.

In each dormitory the beds are arranged against the internal walls, which provides more insulation and also affords a clear view of the dormitory windows and the prospect beyond. The windows operate by a sash, which opens five inches wide so that fresh air can enter but patients cannot fall out. You will see a similar attention to space and fittings as within the day-rooms: an arched wooden door, once unlocked for you, reveals timber floors, plastered walls and an open fireplace. The fireplace is seldom used, as the hot air heating system employed in the day-rooms has also been found sufficient here, while ventilation grates carry the warmth through a system of flues to the connecting corridors. Only in the most severe weather do we find it necessary to light the upstairs fires or to issue extra winter blankets, despite the fact that the ceilings are high and there is a greater allocation upstairs of space per patient.

The dormitories are also lit by coal gas with a pendant lamp hanging from the centre of each room. A lavatory table is provided, incorporating four removable basins, together with soap bowls and towel rails, so that patients may wash or be washed at any time. It can be pushed on castors from bed to bed. Each dormitory also has a commode chair as an alternative to the water closets, while movable screens provide the necessary privacy. Lastly, there is a communal locker in each dormitory so that patients' clothes can be secured at night. These lockers incorporate a bench seat in front of them, on which patients may sit to dress or undress.

An attendant's room overlooks each dormitory. A communication port within each room allows for supervision and also the swift report of any disturbance amongst the patients. Each attendant's room is furnished with a cupboard, shelving and hooks for clothes.

There are slight differences between the dormitories in each block. In the south blocks, the first floor dormitories have adjacent day-rooms, while the second floor is given over entirely to bedrooms. This upper floor accommodates the greatest number of male and female patients: there are six dormitories with twelve beds, and two with fourteen, together with eight single rooms. In the north blocks, both the upper floors are used solely for sleeping, with two large dormitories of fifteen on the male side, and one on the women's, and five single rooms on either side on each floor. The windows in the dormitories are also slightly smaller in the north block, for better safety.

We appreciate that every patient would prefer a single room, but for reasons of economy and security we are able to provide only sixty-three patients with that luxury. Single bedrooms are reserved for patients who are shortly to be discharged on trial, sick in body, or at risk of causing harm to others. These whitewashed bedrooms provide a greater personal space, though there is no direct source of heat, only a grate bringing in warmer air from the corridor outside. Each single room incorporates additional safety features: strong wooden shutters cover the windows when the room is occupied, and the solid oak doors are designed to open outwards only.

Unfortunately, it is not possible to provide light in the single rooms on the north side once the doors and shutters are closed for occupancy, though in the south block the bedrooms include high level, plate glass apertures above the doors to allow in gas light from the corridors.

What our dormitories lack in both individual space and privacy is amply compensated for by their level of comfort. Although a number of asylums make use of iron bed frames, we felt that American birch was warmer, and it allows us to easily build crib bedsteads for agitated patients, while for patients prone to fits we can make a bedstead with four padded sides. We use hair mattresses wherever possible, though coir padding is placed within mattresses for those who may be destructive, or liable to soil themselves at night, as coir pads are harder to rip and more absorbent. Sheets are linen and wool, and are changed every fortnight. A simple white counterpane is placed above the blankets on the female wards, while bright colours and varied patterns are used on the male side. This enables the laundry to keep the linen belonging to the two sides entirely separate.

On the ground and first floors in the north block are rooms fitted out for patients requiring the highest level of safety and security. These are the padded rooms. There are two for patients of each sex. One of the male rooms has its walls covered with hard-wearing leather, while the other three rooms are all treated similarly with India-rubber cloth. The leather room and one of the women's rooms have an additional flooring of linoleum rather than wood, which is easier to clean. These rooms are for occasional use by patients perceived to be at great risk of damaging themselves, other patients or asylum property.

Ward Life

Each floor of a block constitutes at least one ward, and each ward is made up of one or more dormitories with additional single rooms. Within the north block, one ward is reserved for cases suffering from acute signs of active insanity, where staff watchfulness is of great necessity. Some of these refractory cases may benefit from a single room where there is less opportunity for destruction. Similarly, wards are set aside for male and female epileptics, who must be supervised carefully for signs of fits at night.

Incurables or chronic cases make up the rest of the north block, including those who are elderly and unable to fend for themselves.

On the south side, the convalescents or the tranquil and not actively insane can be found recovering. The convalescent wards are the most lavishly decorated. Ample mirrors are available, especially on the female side, so that the women may be given opportunities to tidy themselves and arrange their hair or clothes – an activity which is acknowledged to be good for their health. Cocoa matting is provided to soften the floor boards, while the refinement of the female convalescent day-room is much admired. Colourful ornamental borders bedeck the walls, and the space also doubles as the sewing room, where able seamstresses can work in comfort.

Here the public asylum differs markedly from the private one. In a private asylum, often the only classification is by wealth: so it is the richer patients who have the larger bedrooms and the more sophisticated furnishings, regardless of their symptoms. Similarly, in the private house, patients with all types of diagnoses may mingle in the day-rooms: the manic may disturb the convalescent; the epileptic frighten the melancholic. This is why the private house is less well-equipped for recovery than a public asylum. Allocation by need is not an option to the man running his house for profit.

It is the south block that you will be sent to first, to the ward set aside for new admissions. Unless there are pressing reasons for a move, you will spend your first few weeks here for observation. To a certain extent this ward is unlike the others, in that there is regular movement of patients in and out of it. It is, of necessity, a temporary home, but despite this the facilities of the admissions ward are much like all the others.

In each ward scrupulous arrangements have been made for hygiene and sanitation conveniences, which are always situated at a distance from the sleeping areas and usually separated by a lobby. There is one white porcelain bath and sink on each of the upper south floors, and two porcelain baths on each of the upper north floors. The result is that there is roughly one bath for every twenty-five patients, while there are two water closets on each floor, or roughly one for every twelve patients. The closets are tiled and have a northerly aspect. Within the male side, there are two additional white earthenware urinals placed in the corners of the passageways opposite the closets.

The closets house lavatories constructed on George Jennings' patent flushing mechanism with a high level cistern. These devices are very modern, and you may not have used them before. There has been much debate recently about whether the new water closets are more sanitary than the traditional earth closet. Although our architect ensured a very thorough ventilation in each closet and connecting passageway, with the earth closet there is a greater need still for ventilation; even then, the consequent smell can be most noxious. There is also the additional complication that the earth closet requires emptying at least once a day, which necessitates the carrying of each closet's contents through the building, and is most undesirable.

However, the reliability of the pipes required for water closets has not yet been fully proven. Although our soil pipes are constructed out of earthenware, and sealed with cement, there is still a risk to our wells and water supply by the transportation of foul water to the asylum's filter beds. Nevertheless, public discourse has increasingly favoured the water closet as the most appropriate convenience for residential accommodation, and we have decided to persist with them. We trust you will not find them unsettling. Please be reassured that any possibility of unpleasant overflows or water discharges into the wards has been adequately prevented, and that our architect has taken all precautions possible against sewage gas and its attendant airborne, infectious maladies.

Maladies, and their treatment, will mark the point at which we end our tour. At the far end of each south block you will find the male and female infirmaries. This is the quietest part of the asylum, where patients who are physically unwell might rest and recuperate. There is space here for up to forty patients, mostly in single rooms which, uniquely, have both coal gas lighting and open fires. This is because of the incapacity of those within, and the resulting lower safety risk, as well as the increased level of supervision. Some of the single rooms are also interconnected, allowing an attendant to sleep in one bed next door to a patient requiring particular attention, and the attendants' rooms include a locked medicine chest, which acts as an emergency dispensary.

Every effort has been made towards patient comfort: in addition to the open fires, there are hot water radiators with ornamental gratings; the toilet and bath are placed together in one large, accessible space; cocoa matting is provided to the day-room in each infirmary ward.

In line with advice from the Commissioners in Lunacy, we have also recently begun to segregate infectious patients and those suffering from other ailments. At present, these patients are placed within special corridors where we take all precautions to prevent the air spreading to the rest of the asylum. In the longer term, we have recently gained approval to construct a separate, single-storey building to which these infectious cases will be moved and from which the prevailing wind will shift the air away from our main accommodation.

So ends your view of our facilities. By now, the impression that you should have received is one of cleanliness, healthiness and industry. There is a regular programme of whitewashing of the walls and ceilings in the wards and the day-rooms, such that every year parts of the asylum are always freshly painted, and the exterior wood and metalwork are constantly maintained.

Our asylum is a cheerful proposition. This befits the general view held by most right-thinking people that the patients deserve the best that can be afforded to people in their position. During a recent visit by the local bishop, he remarked that he was 'struck by the air of brightness and cheerfulness' in the wards and 'with the perfect order prevailing throughout the house.'

Clothing and Personal Possessions

Before we leave you on the admissions ward, our remaining task is to deal with your personal possessions. It is not always possible for you to take personal items into the asylum, partly because of your own illness and partly due to the communal nature of the institution; an object which may be harmless in one pair of hands can become dangerous in others. To a certain extent, what you are able to keep depends on which ward you are placed after your movement from the admissions ward; but even then, the assessment will be made with your fellow occupants in mind as much as your own needs.

Patients often like to bring personal photographs or letters on to the wards and we will generally try to guarantee an element of individuality. Other keepsakes, either ornamental such as jewellery, or practical such as braces or cufflinks are not often permitted. Every item that you cannot take will be securely stored in the institution, though with your permission your possessions may also be returned to your family. Items taken onto the wards can be kept in the clothing locker.

You may have noticed on your tour that very few patients wear their own clothes. Generally speaking, the asylum wardrobe is to be preferred as this makes all patients equal and the washing easier for the laundry staff, but we have no objection to special items being provided by your family; indeed, for many patients a favourite hat or shawl may be some comfort as a reminder of their domestic life. You will also see some patients who are always dressed in their own clothes, as some private patients (or, more usually, their families) prefer to maintain this privilege. The same privilege may also be afforded those who are shortly to be discharged on trial, assuming they have funds to purchase a suitable set of clothing. But the vast majority of patients possess a hard-wearing, modest yet practical asylum uniform, and you too will be expected to wear it.

Before we opened, fabric samples were requested from a number of other asylums with the aim of procuring cloth that, while meeting our strict financial considerations, was also designed to benefit the comfort, appearance and health of the patients. The clothes are of heavy, durable material so that they may last for a worthwhile period of time, and are also designed for year-round use so that they will not be too warm in summer, yet provide the requisite insulation in winter. You will be issued with underwear, outer garments and night clothes sufficient to provide for the weekly changeovers of clothes.

Underwear is of linen. Drawers, which are knee-length, are changed once a week, as are nightshirts, while socks and stockings are changed twice a week. Similarly, the linen shirts and blouses – a pale grey calico – are changed twice a week. For patients who are minded to sleep without clothes, additional blankets can be provided. Pullovers of Guernsey wool are available too, if required.

For men, the usual outerwear is a three-piece suit of brown tweed, with a similar suit of bright pilot blue for Sundays and holidays. The tweed for the jackets and waistcoats can be fashioned in a small range of differing patterns. Trousers are generally plain and are available with fly or, for those patients desirous of behaving in an indecent manner, a version is produced with a flap; this can be securely fastened to the waistcoat and released by staff when necessary. A tweed cap is available should extra protection be required from sun or rain, and overcoats will be provided if the weather is excessively grave or the patient elderly and infirm.

Women patients are given two dresses of linsey – a rather coarse cloth of wool and linen intertwined, but one that is hard-wearing, economical and warm. There are winter colours in dark shades of brown, blue or green; while in summer a similar dress is provided with a coloured print. Dresses for the most chronic patients will be hemmed up, so that they do not fall below the ankle: a chronic patient is unlikely to lift their hem above the ground, which can be a source of much damage to the cloth in poor weather.

Where possible, decoration is provided, as plain dresses are not becoming to most women. Efforts are made to encourage some patients to take up crochet and to introduce lace effects to their clothing at the wrists and neck. Petticoats are offered as an additional layer between the female under and outer-garments. Women also have the option of a cream tartan shawl, which gives a group of female patients out walking a most picturesque appearance. In the summer, straw hats with a variety of coloured ribbons are available to provide protection from the solar glare, with those worn by the more agitated patients secured with a strap and buckle. Mature patients can be provided with a cloth cap.

Generally, outer garments are intended to last for about two years. Destructive patients are liable to be given garments which have been re-sewn or patched together from items handed down from other patients, and those who have a tendency to drool may also find their clothes protected by an apron or a pinafore. Please be aware that outerwear is usually fashioned on more generous sizes so that, as much as possible, one size will fit any new admission. We aim to give a broad outline of shape, but do not be too disheartened if you find the fit unfashionable or unsuited to your figure. There is usually a wider range of underwear available, so that stocking, socks or drawers should fit comfortably, whatever the necessary compromises of the other garments.

For the workers, or those permitted to go on long walks outside, leather boots are provided; while cloth shoes suffice – with leather galoshes for wet weather – for those who remain indoors or whose external world extends only to the airing courts. All boots have buckles for fastening, with buttons for the shoes; laces are best avoided for the melancholy. Working men and women additionally receive a pair of cloth slippers to be worn in the evenings or at activities such as dancing.

The Cost of Your Stay

All of these facilities: heat, light, food, bedding and clothing are provided by the local poor rate. Around thirteen shillings a week is allocated for your care. Do not forget to thank the ratepayers for their beneficence in providing you with care at no expense to yourself. It is, of course, now an accepted tenet of our civilised society that those who have the means should support those with no hope of providing for themselves. Nevertheless, the sacrifices of the ratepayer must not be taken for granted.

That is not to say that it is impossible to enhance your stay in any way. While you may be without means – and your arrival here is likely proof of that – your family or friends may be granted the indulgence of providing little things for you. There is no system of patient accounts as you might find in a private house or a government asylum, but the occasional book or other treat might be passed on to you if it is considered safe to do so. If you or your friends truly wish some freedom to be allowed within the bounds of your position here, then there is always the option of transferring your case to the register of private patients.

Chapter 4

Diagnosis

The path by which you have arrived here has been constructed by well-intentioned persons, though individuals who are unlikely to possess expertise in the diseases of the human mind. It is our duty to test their conclusions and to form a diagnosis, and we shall do so through both inquiry and observation. Once you are settled on the admissions ward, one of the medical officers will conduct an interview with you. They will make notes on physical matters such as your skin and hair colour; the state of your tongue and your appetite; matters relating to your reproductive organs; the responsiveness of your senses; and to the regularity and consistency of your bowel movements. There will also be questions about your emotions, how you feel at that moment and what symptoms you are experiencing.

There are a number of predisposing causes of insanity which we are bound to investigate by inquiry. These relate mostly to your own history and that of your family members, for example, the condition of your parents at the time of your birth may provide clues as to your current state. If they were suffering from some illness or intoxication at the moment of conception, then this may have been passed on to you. Similarly, the act of labour may have resulted in damage to you or to the mother who nursed you. It is a well-established fact that childbirth is performed less easily amongst the women of developed nations, and many commentators argue that our own industrial improvement has made a severe impact on the prevalence of insanity.

Of equal weight, at least, are your own experiences during the critical periods of life, be that teething, puberty, sexual maturity or, for women, the additional risks arising from pregnancy, lactation and cessation of the menstrual flow. Physical triggers for insanity can also be found through illnesses, including fevers, head injuries or over-exposure to the sun.

Although it is sometimes suggested that the female of the species is more physically predisposed to insanity, it is also acknowledged that proportionately, the male is more at risk of succumbing to disease, as a result of the far greater agitation from moral causes afforded during the average man's daily life. Partly this is due to choice of profession: the Commissioners in Lunacy's reports regularly comment on the high levels of insanity amongst ex-members of the armed forces, as well as gentlemen of superior learning, or those involved in trade or finance. It is also due to the pressure on the male to maintain a suitable level of income to ensure his family's security, and assert his own professional power to carve out a position in life.

Hereditary factors were once regarded as playing an important role in a diagnosis of insanity, though this presumption is increasingly being challenged. Nevertheless, the question will be raised, but not in such a manner as to cause you or your family embarrassment. The same is true of questions about your consumption of liquor. Tact is one of the principal duties of our medical men. Nor do we make assumptions about your illness. Our initial questions are a chance for you to tell us how you are feeling, and whether anything is troubling you. Please do not feel obliged to answer any question that makes you feel uncomfortable. We shall lead you gently through the pathways of your life history, and thrust open no door that you wish to remain closed.

There are, of course, also ways for us to observe you, and these will not cause you any disquiet, indeed, you may not be aware of them at all. While some men can be judged insane by conversation alone, for others it is by their conduct that diagnosis will be made. To a certain extent, such conduct is likely to have been remarked upon in the paperwork that accompanied you: most physicians will draw attention to a want of order in your actions or personal appearance. Some patients prefer to clothe themselves in fanciful costumes or wear nothing at all; sometimes their bodies have swollen through the intake of food, yet others respond to the act of digestion with revulsion; sometimes language is missing, while in others it is excessive; there may be an unnatural fondness for a particular article in your possession; and at times a patient's range of facial expressions is enough to suggest a particular illness.

Our interview and observations will, in due course, inform your allocation to a permanent ward. Influencing factors include the duration of the illness – for a chronic case is always less hopeful than an acute one – as well as any tendency to behave in either a noisy, unclean, violent or suicidal manner. Desire to work is another factor, as is a desire to engage in offensive habits. All these elements add up to a picture of what current level of supervision may be required. Generally, patients of similar behaviours are grouped together, so that those with a propensity to disrupt their fellows are at least together with those too cocooned within their own annoyances or pay them any heed.

We appreciate that classification is impossible beyond a simple statement of your symptoms. Insanity is a most peculiar state and defies attempts to contain it within one label or another. Modern alienists recognise this, and your diagnosis will present you only as experiencing one of a few, widely accepted conditions. The greater proportion of patients – as many as eight in every ten – will usually be considered to have mania or dementia, while of the remainder, around half are considered melancholic. These are the principal diagnoses of lunacy, though others are available.

A smaller sub-group of our patients are not really lunatics at all: these are the mentally defective, the idiots and imbeciles who were born lacking part of their mental capacities. Members of all these groups can be found on any one ward.

Mania

The poor wretch raving, oblivious in his madness, is a traditional representation of insanity. Acute mania is easy for the layman to understand, for it acts as a shaft of moonlight directly illuminating the lunatic from his saner cousins. The behaviour associated with mania is distinctive, and the disease brings with it a passion that is uncontrollable and prolonged.

Many sufferers of mania will barely sleep, unable to rest long enough for darkness to quell the turbulence within their minds; while conscious, they tend to speak franticly, spewing out words and making wild gestures almost without cease. Their torrent of ideas, noise or actions informs the physician of his patient's state. Language may be fanciful, foul or free-flowing; words flee from the pen; bedding or clothing may be ripped and cast aside. The manic tirelessly seek satisfaction, yet can find none. No imposter would try to fake acute mania for they would exhaust themselves in the attempt.

This state of excitement chiefly characterises the disease. Amongst our patients is E.B., 34, who is suffering from an acute attack of mania. She is a recently-widowed housewife with three young children, and was brought in after trying to commit suicide, first by biting herself and then by banging her head against the wall of the workhouse ward. She talks constantly, throws herself about and tears at any fabric within reach.

Sometimes an acute attack of mania can be deduced very promptly. A quickened pulse may be used as evidence for its arrival, while often the appetite is increased. Once mania has settled and become chronic, then the symptoms of an acute attack are joined by others peculiar to each case. J.T., a 29-year-old schoolteacher has been suffering from mania for over five years. On the ward you will find him talking incoherently to himself and making incessant gestures. His bowels are uncontrolled and he is liable to break things in the day-room. He has also developed a voracious appetite for grass and, more worryingly, coal, and if left to himself outside he will forage for either delicacy. We have found that he becomes calm only when listening to music or singing.

There is no guarantee that delusions may be present in mania for, though you may be restless, your mind is not necessarily distorted. You may dance, or sing, or fight in a futile attempt to dissolve your energies, rather than because you are hearing music or because imaginary devils are upon you. Nevertheless, the result for sufferers is the same level of disorientation as may be experienced by a delusion. At the extremity of mania there is some connection with acute melancholia, and it is not uncommon for the physician to determine a patient as manic with melancholic tendencies, or the reverse. Suicidal patients are often considered to be suffering from mania, even if they are in a melancholic phase. The other disease associated with mania is the general paralysis of the insane (further discussed below), which may include a manic phase during its progression. A paralytic maniac will calm down within a month or so of onset; the illness of the true maniac will continue far beyond such a point.

Mania may take other forms that stop short of such extravagant behaviour, and in this modern age diagnosis is subject to a process of constant refinement and distinction. We now recognise mania regarding a particular aspect of normal functions and urges: insanitary habits, such as the consumption of faeces or urine; an inappropriate libido; gorging on food or vomiting. Similarly, compulsions considered morally wrong may find themselves described as manic if the individual is consumed by them and unable to stop their behaviour: compulsive thieving, fire-starting or erotic tendencies are all sub-classes of the disease. Observation will allow us to conclude whether such appetites and perversions have become indecorous.

In a significant minority of cases mania is found to be relapsing but recurrent. Many patients have left asylum care as rational men and women and contentedly rejoined their previous lives, only for another attack to occur, followed by the inevitable return journey to the asylum. Hysteria is a prime example of such cases, where a female crisis can quickly bring about a new onslaught of disease. J.B., a middle-aged field-worker has had many attacks of mania during the past ten years. When she is unwell, she sleeps barely an hour at night in the dormitory, while she shouts continuously during the day. When she is better, she is able to work on her ward or in the laundry; but these periods of good health never last long. For patients like this, the wide range of potentially exciting causes render it very difficult to predict with any certainty whether a temporary recovery will become permanent. All too often, respite is brief.

Eventually, the maniac is so exhausted that few vestiges of the self remain. In this, the raving madman differs from the sufferer whose mania takes on more subtle forms. These subtleties are often assigned to the epithet of monomania, and we will discuss them under that name.

Dementia

The concept of dementia is equally easy to understand: it is one of loss. The capacity that once existed for rational thought is now compromised in some way. Unlike an idiot or imbecile, who has never enjoyed that capacity, the sufferer of dementia is able to feel the lack of the facility they formerly had. Thus the demented may act as an infant in knowledge, actions or responses but they are most certainly adult, and once operated in an adult form.

Sometimes sufferers from dementia are aware of the advance of their condition. The disease can be slow to take hold, progressing gently over a number of years. The patient may experience occasional forgetfulness or incoherence for long periods before it becomes a noticeable problem. The unfortunate sufferer is then able to appreciate their descent into the slough of nature's vacuum. Once the disease has fully taken hold, patients will forget even such details as their own names and how to care for themselves; they seem increasingly dreamlike and distracted. They have regressed to a state of nativity, though lacking the purpose of enquiry that is found in the young. Often patients relive their own childhood emotions, so that the contented child becomes a placid and friendly patient; while one who experienced unhappiness may find their adult mind becoming filled with anger.

On our male side there are dementia sufferers such as J.N., aged 61, who was a general labourer in his previous life. Now he does not know where he is, or what year we are in. He knows that he has children, but he no longer believes they are his. Instead he paces the ward anxiously, convinced that he has committed a crime and asking the staff whether he is to be hanged. On the female side you may meet S.J.A., 52, who worked as a dressmaker and for many years cared for her elderly mother alone. She recently attempted to strangle herself with a bandage and was removed here. Prior to that point, she had suddenly begun to neglect her household chores, to collect rubbish from the streets and to fill her cupboards with it. Here, her loss of memory has become apparent; she takes no notice of life on the ward, and struggles to find answers to questions put to her.

We will always probe for symptoms such as these, and it has long been held that the use of numbers and letters can assist in diagnosing cases of dementia. Should we fear that you may be suffering from the condition, we may ask you questions based on the recognition of numbers, or whether you can write a simple sentence. Such abstract questions draw out the loss of memory in the dementia patient.

Sadly, some demented persons suffer from disagreeable symptoms. Many patients forget how to care for themselves or to perform the most basic routines of hygiene, while the disease is also attended by a general relaxation of the muscles. Patients lose control of their bladder or bowels, or become prone to the vices of masturbation and exhibitionism. As a result, dementia patients usually require a higher degree of care than other lunatics.

In some cases of dementia affecting younger persons it is not memory but judgement that is impaired. The enfeeblement of the intellect wears down the patient's understanding of what is real and what is imagined. Delusions are present though without the extreme agitation associated with mania. These cases are often found to have their origin in a particular event of happiness or sorrow, which can be recounted with unusual clarity by the patient. J.H., for example, is an ex-soldier whose disease came on when he was 33 years of age. He says that during his service he was put into a black hole together with a roaring lion. Throughout his time here he has become increasingly still and silent. At first he would do a little scrubbing in the wards, though he complained at night that a great snake was placed in the bed beside him. Now he is listless and vacant. He sits all day, performing imaginary actions, picking things up from the floor, the table or the air and then eating them. He is prone to wet himself or soil his clothing and must be washed regularly.

Dementia such as this is sometimes perceived to follow either mania or melancholia, and a firm diagnosis may not be made for some months, until an acute attack of the other symptoms has subsided.

Melancholia

Melancholia was, for many years, seen as the twin of mania. It shares a similar emotional intensity to the latter condition, though rather than inspiring excessive gaiety and energy, melancholia gifts its victims only despondency, sloth and fear. A sufferer may become withdrawn and unable to cope with life; they may seek solitude or even their own destruction. Essentially, not only are they cheerless in mind but the mind itself is consumed intently with the fact of its own cheerlessness; melancholia is, therefore, as exhausting a disease as mania.

It has often been theorised that melancholia stems solely from the moral causes of insanity: that grief, anxieties and reverses of fortune are the trigger. The disappointment then clings to the person and they cannot free themselves of it. In this, melancholia differs from the normal passing phase of sorrow. Melancholia grips a person until their will is lost. W.S.'s case would seem to illustrate this: he is 45 and has suffered a series of reverses in life. He was married for twenty years and had several children, but all save one died young. When his wife died two years ago, W.S. suddenly lost all his energy and strength. He could no longer be persuaded to work, and his surviving daughter felt obliged to hide his razor as he was so frequently asking for it. Now he resides here.

Nevertheless, it is rare indeed that a case of melancholia has a sudden onset. The disease generally has a lengthy progression, and at first may seem no more than a slight exaggeration of a patient's underlying character. It is only with the passage of time that one can see the melancholic's thoughts drawn back constantly towards the source of gloom, as if he were a shadow continually trying to escape the pull of the dark. It is at this point that delusions or hallucinations can be observed in the conversation of many a melancholic patient, while the most severe cases become almost paralysed and unable even to speak.

H.T. is a 50-year-old housewife. When she came to us her hair was thick, grey and matted, and her clothes were filthy. She had evidently neglected herself for some time. If you see her on the ward now, you will find her both depressed and nervous, worried for her personal safety and awaiting what she believes to be her reckoning. She says that she has stolen many things and begs to be taken to the police so that they might arrest her. She looks distracted as she waits for the officers to arrive and spirit her away. She is a woman at a certain time of life, and this may well be the underlying cause of her desperation. The acute onset of her illness was brought about, however, by an article she read in the newspaper about the Shipton rail disaster, when so many passengers on the Great Western Railway lost their lives. She is convinced that she caused the tragedy and for this reason she believes her suffering is inevitable.

Melancholia such as this may be accurately diagnosed through observation. The grip of sadness leads to a stooped and drooping posture, engulfed in slow and painful movement, while the face is bereft of any sparks of life. Sufferers of melancholia are additionally by far the most aware of any member of our patient cohort. They are able to describe both the causes and the symptoms of their disease, while they can also anticipate the foreboding of an attack and perceive the inevitability of each setback. If you wish to articulate your unworthy life, your affliction with a deadly ailment, or your suspicion that some person or institution has set out to ruin you, then we will be happy to listen to you expound your tale of woe.

An interview with a melancholic is therefore likely to be lengthy. While the maniac is too flighty to focus on conversation, we can ask a depressed patient about their health, their friends and family, their expectations, their spiritual or emotional beliefs, and expect a full response. We will observe their rest too, for the restorative powers of sleep are often denied to the melancholy, for whom a silent night provides space for further brooding. S.C. is one of our nocturnally troubled patients. She is the wife of a cellarman and mother to a young child. She has exhausted herself with suckling her infant, lost her faith and abandoned herself to the hopelessness of existence. She seeks only to bring about her own destruction, and it is at night and in the morning when this suicidal impulse is strongest; her mood lightens quickly once she begins work.

S.C. demonstrates another notable feature of the melancholic: the ability to live within a system of sadness without it having an obvious impact on daily life. Even the delusions of the melancholic may be faced inward, so that they do not affect those around him. Since the flame of hope has been extinguished, a melancholic's false beliefs do not necessarily lead to any subsequent action. As a result, the melancholic can successfully disguise their insanity, and may even deny it if confronted by it. Patience is the virtue of the physician who works with melancholia.

Monomania

As research into the nature of insanity continues, so alienists have begun to uncover more conditions. It is to this group of newly identified illnesses that the epithet of monomania belongs.

Monomania always results in a most particular delusion: one solitary, irrational falsehood is taken as a truth upon which the disordered mind builds further schemes and actions. This fantasy building is of a most logical nature, but it is unstable because the foundations are wrong. The nature of the initial delusion will vary, but it usually places the patient in a position where he must act either to bring about some great event or to prevent one. An element of conspiracy is also often present. Thus, a patient may feel themselves quite right to warn society of impending doom – an act that any responsible citizen might consider – but if that source of doom is imaginary, then the patient can do nothing but harm in pursuing his quest.

At its most creative, monomania can include full sensory hallucinations, such that serpents might be seen to lurk beneath the floors or spectres to be perched above the roofs; equally, the illness may fixate itself on real beings, who can then find themselves at risk. Whatever the nature of the delusion, it will be localised, and is unlikely to cross over into other aspects of the patient's life.

Consider the case of F.S., an ex-soldier of 37 years who has served in India. He has monomania of suspicion: he believes that sexual irritants are being placed in beer, that both he and his wife took this contaminated drink, and that persons unknown continue to poison him. To escape his persecutors F.S. believes his only option is to flee to America, where he will be safe. He is wary of the asylum food. However, if he can be diverted from his passion, the patient is happy and content, working in the kitchen garden and apparently enjoying his occupation.

F.B. is a middle-aged farmer who has become obsessed with his financial affairs. He has lately encountered money troubles, and now believes that he is entitled to an allowance from the Duke of Cambridge. He also believes that he has been wronged by his brother, who obtained a court judgement against him for a payment owed. He intended to shoot his brother but, finding him not at home, shot one of his cows instead. Ever since he came here it has become apparent how this delusion spreads. If spoken to today, he will assure you that his debts are partly due to his investment in a fictitious grammar school, to his spotting defects in the old Westminster Bridge, and to the building of this asylum, the construction of which he believes results from a dispute between him and his neighbours. Yet, on all these matters his speech is utterly coherent, and he is polite, orderly and industrious; in many ways the model patient.

The monomaniac is thus a man whose insanity is only ever partial. To the layman, the patient appears no less sane than his neighbour, as he is able to converse on a number of topics and to act rationally in relation to them. His intellect and reasoning seem undimmed by illness, and it is only by touching on the nature of the delusion itself that the disease becomes apparent. In consequence, many months of careful observation may be necessary to prove the disease. Equally, it might often seem that an otherwise rational person could be challenged about the basis of such a limited delusion, yet the monomaniac is by their very nature unable to disprove it. Their legs may not resemble wood, but that does not mean that if you cut them they would not be wood inside.

Moral Insanity

Like monomania, moral insanity is a modern concept. It is a condition where the patient's powers of reason work efficiently, and it is often considered to be a disease free from all delusion. Instead, the symptoms of the disease are based around deficiencies of moral sense. Reason has not been lost but has instead been perverted. Of course, variations in morality will be found amongst all men. Although as a society we try to attain virtue and avoid sin, it is inevitable that as individuals we may take subtly different views about what sort of behaviours are normal practice in these pursuits. Where the sufferer from moral insanity differs is that his behaviour is of such great variance from the rest of society that it becomes intolerable.

The current medical conclusion is that the patient's will has been subsumed by a desire. Sometimes a patient labours under an irresistible impulse, unable to prevent their actions, however harmful. In other cases all emotional normality is jettisoned, and the sufferer acts without the usual fear of consequence. This renders them reckless, and the result can be inappropriate behaviour that is merely alarming or more obviously destructive. The erotic vanity of an old woman apt to colour her face and adorn herself in tinsel may be unnerving, but the unchecked libido of a young man can be a source of danger. Both individuals might be considered to be suffering from moral insanity, and both might be suitable cases for treatment.

Some form of callousness, masked by plausibility, is a typical feature of moral insanity. Friends and family of such patients often put up with their perverted behaviour for years, constantly reassured by the sufferer that no wrong has been done, before they find that their companion can no longer be managed or that the local magistrates have become involved. For the morally insane are able to commit atrocities and then justify them, removing the blame elsewhere. They may also express themselves seized with the wish to change their ways, while still working to subvert the very cures on which they claim salvation.

Moral insanity is perhaps the hardest of our acknowledged illnesses of the mind to diagnose. These cases are also rare: the only one in memory here was A.H., a young woman who was a compulsive thief. Though she was admitted to our care it was clear that mentally, she suffered no apparent defects and she was discharged within weeks of her arrival. Her case relates to characteristics of personality rather than identifiable illness. Cases like this have led to a further classification of 'moral imbecility' being considered by alienists.

Neither prolonged conversation nor physical observation is guaranteed to bring about a clear diagnosis of moral insanity, as for much of the time it is a concealed disease, becoming apparent only when an outburst can be witnessed. Because of this we are reluctant to diagnose it unless certain that there is no other underlying condition.

General Paralysis

The general paralysis of the insane is usually considered a disease in its own right, even if its early symptoms can sometimes be confused with other states of lunacy, meaning that it is often undiagnosed until its final stages. What causes general paralysis is still a mystery to physicians, though it is worth noting that the disease is seldom, if ever seen in those of less than 30 years of age. It is an adult affliction with distinct physical symptoms.

These symptoms can sometimes appear subtle to the untrained eye, but gradually all tend towards a loss of function and co-ordination of the muscles. Speech may be affected and the paralytic patient slurs or droops like a drunken wretch; reflexes are gradually lost; and added to the rolling speech and gait is an inability to swallow or control the bowels. Sores may appear on any part of the body and are impossible to heal. These are the later stages of the disease, and a full paralysis is quite obvious by its physical effects.

We must warn you that the prognosis in such cases is not good. J.Hr., a police constable, was sent to us five months ago with a vacant gaze, listlessness and indistinct speech. This dullness has increased along the lines described above and it is apparent that his death is close at hand.

Feigned Insanity

It is our duty to be sure that your case is one of genuine insanity. It is rare, but occasionally we encounter patients who evidently have the desire to be thought of as insane, though in truth they are not. This is a particular route taken by some felons who wish to avoid the more exacting rigours of the gaol, though it is also a ruse that some tramps use to escape harsh conditions on the road.

Fortunately, the sane man stands out amongst the rank and file of lunatics. An ex-patient, J.Ht. was admitted having been spotted loitering outside a bank. In the local cells he claimed at once that he was aide-de-camp for the Crown Prince of Prussia, as well as the son of King George III and the Governor of the Bank of England. But these statements were entirely random, and did not tend towards any subsequent belief or action. In contrast, each lunatic has a particular system to his madness, a system that the sane are quite unable to replicate. J.Ht. was an imposter, and information was soon received to that effect from a neighbouring asylum. When confronted, J.Ht. admitted his malingering tendency and explained that when he gets a little drink he 'goes wrong'.

Amentia, or Idiocy and Imbecility

Amentia, or absence of mind, is not a disease as such; rather, it is a state of development. Sufferers are those whose intellectual faculties were never fully established – reason has not been lost because it was never there. Patients affected by amentia are usually described as idiots, imbeciles or the mentally defective, and the condition itself is wont to be classified according to the degree of helplessness from which the patient suffers. The true idiot finds himself unable to function on his own: incapable of either gaining sustenance or reproduction. Some idiots are also mute, deaf or blind. As one moves up the scale the higher forms of imbecile are capable of eating, bathing and dressing themselves; while some even converse in simple terms.

At this higher end of amentia, many patients may have happily taken care of themselves, held down basic work, and displayed a range of emotions. T.S. is one such example. Now aged 44, he was born the illegitimate son of an agricultural labourer and for years he had found seasonal work, interspersed with periods in the workhouse. Though he can only answer 'yes' or 'no' to any question put to him, he has managed to get by. His removal here was due to a sudden inclination to commit unnatural offences with other workhouse inmates. We have found him hard to manage, as he wets and soils himself, and is liable to annoy the other patients by shouting noisily at them or by trying to steal their food at mealtimes.

However, we will not give up on his recovery merely because he is one of our more challenging patients. Dr Down's recent work at Earlswood Asylum on Mongolian syndrome has proved there is the potential for such patients to benefit from the asylum regime, to take part in activities and be trained for employment. This suggests that there is little reason why some amentia sufferers should not make their own way in society. That men and women like this end up here instead is probably because a source of work is denied them or their family is not able to support them. They have probably also displayed some petty behaviour that makes them unsuitable for the workhouse.

Many idiots can be diagnosed by visual observation. They have large heads, malformed faces or disproportionate limbs. Similarly, epilepsy can provide a clue to idiocy, as each fit observed is liable to damage the brain and render it less productive. E.H., an 11-year-old girl, has been an epileptic idiot since birth. She was supposed for years to be also deaf and dumb, but we have found her capable of uttering a few words even though she does not understand what is said to her. She is powerless to wash or feed herself and needs help with both procedures. When she was first admitted she was violent too and would throw her clothes around, though over time she has become a little calmer and is being taught to sew.

It perhaps seems odd that idiots and imbeciles are considered to be suitable asylum patients, given that their conditions cannot be alleviated. The reason for this is that the condition of idiocy has long been given over to the alienists to study. Nevertheless, the differences between lunatics and the disabled are widely noted and there is increasing encouragement to give them alternative arrangements according to their different needs.

Chapter 5

Staff

For the purpose of your stay, the staff at the asylum can be neatly grouped into two communities: those whom you will see around on a daily basis; and those who work behind the scenes. Within both communities is an order of command and a series of duties carefully defined so that everyone may know his task. Stepping outside those duties, or performing them incorrectly, is considered a noteworthy misdemeanour. There is also a natural division between the different classes of staff, reflecting their rank within the asylum.

Ultimate power rests, of course, in the committee of visitors, but as these men are unable to offer more than the occasional period of time, they must, of necessity, delegate the responsibility for running the asylum to their appointees, and here the true hierarchy begins. We shall consider each of them in turn: officers, attendants, and servants.

The Asylum Officers

The Medical Superintendent

As any army needs its general, so too does the asylum require its superintendent. For the superintendent directs all that goes on – he is the head of medicine, as well as of staff management – and his control extends to every aspect of life in the institution. He is by some distance the best paid member of staff (let us suggest a salary in the region of £400 per annum), and also enjoys a generous allowance of six weeks' leave. He is appointed solely by the committee of visitors – from whom he must seek permission for any absence – and acts as their representative during daily operations.

Asylum superintendents are very rare birds. They combine a forensic aptitude for scientific analysis with the decision-making skills of the brightest administrators. It is a given that, when appointed, they should already be of high standing in their profession: a member of one of the colleges of surgeons or physicians and a former student of one of the universities. In addition, they are highly practical exponents of the art of the mind-doctor. Superintendents have first to hone their skills as assistant medical officers before they can be considered suitable to run an asylum. This does not mean that they are necessarily aged, for a medical man's career can progress quickly. Our first superintendent was appointed while in his early thirties and the present one assumed control at the age of 29.

The superintendent commands respect, but is also able to listen carefully to both his staff and patients. He exercises a benevolent control over his institution based on experience of his situation and a confidence in its handling. Yet this is not an arrogant or inaccessible man, and you will see him every day in his smart suit as he makes his rounds. He is also expected to make unannounced visits to the wards at any time of day or night so that he can see that all is well. On any of these occasions you may ask to speak to him, and he shall be happy to hear you; equally, you must obey his instructions.

One of the ills resolved by the modern asylum is the previous tendency for superintendents to undertake external paid work. Often these men were in private practice, and saw their public income as merely another part of their personal receipts, to be treated as with any other contract. This merger of the public purse with private business led to poor medical standards, and patient care became a barrier to profit rather than a central tenet. The filth and restraint in which many patients found themselves was detailed in the 1844 report by Parliament which led to the reforms of the following year. The lawmakers insisted that the modern superintendent devotes the whole of his time to the office from which the ratepayers expect so much.

The care and treatment of his patients must be the primary concern for any superintendent. Thus the provision of comfort, accommodation, occupation and amusement are all ultimately laid at his door. While he may delegate some matters to his supporting officers, it should be remembered that there is a medical element to every aspect of hospital care, even the lines on the cricket pitch and the linen on the beds.

Each morning, the superintendent will arrive at his desk to find a series of reports from his officers and senior attendants, describing anything of note that should be queried or examined on his rounds. As well as the condition of all patients, both male and female, the superintendent is additionally responsible for the cleanliness and presentation of the male wards, and this is a further object of his daily inspection.

The devotion to duty required can lead some superintendents to attempt control of every detail in their charge. The tale of our first superintendent is a salutary one. He was appointed as the building was still under construction, and made many helpful suggestions as to its fittings and fixtures. But in time this focus on the minutiae of his empire became his undoing.

He had always been an obsessive character, a lifelong bachelor, whose circle of friends dwindled as the years wore on and he became ever more anxious about his work. He was reluctant to take holidays and seldom was seen at meetings with his professional colleagues. Gradually, his standards were set so high that none could achieve them, and after fifteen years of trying to fulfil his exacting strictures two of his senior staff decided that they could work with him no longer. They resigned. His own health broke down while he tried to recruit their successors, and he died exhausted some five months later.

This demonstrates the strain that is placed upon those in high office. Here is the man of whom all requests must be made. The superintendent interviews patients who wish to see him, or who are presented as suitable for discharge on trial. More unpleasantly, so too falls to him the duty of carrying out post mortems on patients who pass away while in our care.

It is the superintendent also who decides where each patient should be placed within the asylum, and no movement between the wards is undertaken without his express order. The superintendent assesses whether any patient requires a change in diet and updates the attendants on the numbers in the wards and the rations to allow. He oversees the keeping of records, of movements in or out of the asylum or other incidents, of staff appointments and behaviour, details of receipts, expenditures and stock; and these are collated and in due course form the basis of his reports to the committee of visitors.

The superintendent is additionally the link between the patients and life outside the asylum. He is obliged to decide whether letters written by patients may be forwarded or, alternatively, received by them; to keep patients' friends and family informed of any concerns or the sickness of a patient. He is assisted in his work by the proximity of his abode, which is adjacent to the asylum block. Thus he is always close at hand and able to deal directly with any need. His omnipresence provides reassurance that a familiar face will be continually present during your stay.

The Chaplain

You may have encountered many different characters of priest; those who hold strongly to one or other interpretation of the scriptures, and whose wish is that others may have their eyes opened to this particular interpretation; some for whom the words of God lay heavy, like a sombre beam that supports the soul; and others who believe that only they can channel the mysteries of the divinity.

Such men are not to be found in an asylum, where propensities to fanaticism, guilt or exclusivity are not useful traits. Rather, our chaplain provides a broad church and he can also raise spirits and turn his hand to many secular pastimes without brooding on the delicacies of religion. He plays cricket and helps out with the entertainments. He is one of us.

Any asylum chaplain will have graduated from the universities of Oxford, Cambridge, Edinburgh or London, before being ordained in holy orders. Like all the officers his work at the asylum is his only calling, though he may also be found teaching scripture at the local village school, where the children of our attendants and servants receive their own instruction. Within the clergy the post has a junior air, and as a result the chaplain is often a novice embarking on his career. This leads to a rather high turnover of chaplains, as the role compares unfavourably with the benefits available to a rector, and twice already we have lost our clerics to better offers from a local parish.

Our present chaplain has previously been a curate at various places across the country, including a rural poor law union. He joined us from a church in Hackney, where he had published some works about the area's local history – an achievement for which he was made a fellow of the Royal Historical Society. We hope that he turns out to be a greater success than his predecessor, a married man with seven children, who had been given a second chance after he formed a most unwise extra-marital liaison with the village school mistress. Following months of intrigue the pair eloped to Uxbridge, returning, allegedly contrite, a few days later. Relieved of his parish duties and sent to us instead, he disappeared last autumn without notice. It transpired that he had gambled his way into substantial debt. When one last horse failed to triumph, he resolved to escape his creditors by boarding the next boat for Montevideo. He has not been heard of since.

That these things can happen demonstrates how the chaplain exists somewhat separately from much of what goes on in the asylum. Although nominally under the control of the superintendent, the role of chaplain has much independence, and he is in some respects of equal standing to the senior man. The chaplain is the only other officer granted the maximum of six weeks' leave, for example, and he is also second (if a rather distant second) in salary only to the superintendent. This enhanced standing reflects the other-worldly qualities of spiritual direction; it would be a rash superintendent indeed who would interfere with the content of morning prayers or Divine Service.

The chaplain's key responsibility, of course, is of pastoral care for his flock. This care extends to staff as well as patients and also to former patients out on trial, if it is practicable for him to visit them. You will see the chaplain regularly around the asylum, as in addition to the fixed daily and weekly services he is also at liberty to hold prayers in any of the wards or day-rooms at a time of his choosing. This is of particular benefit to patients who may be unable to attend chapel due to the symptoms of their illness or poor physical health. In fact, the chaplain is instructed to pay special attention to the sick or dying, and he visits the infirmary ward on most days.

The other principal element to his pastoral care is that of education. The chaplain is our schoolmaster and librarian. He purchases newspapers, periodicals and literature for the patients, adding to some 600 books available within the institution. He promotes reading and undertakes such elementary education as he feels may benefit his cohort in writing and arithmetic alongside religious knowledge. You may also find that the chaplain, on one of his regular visits to the wards, may decide to make a presentation on some secular topic, such as natural history or the story of foreign nations, or to engage you in some improving conversation.

The Assistant Medical Officer

The role of assistant medical officer suggests a more junior post than that of superintendent, and it is true that many medical officers arrive at asylums fresh from their university or professional training. After a period of schooling, or the more traditional apprenticeship to an experienced physician, this post can be seen as a first stepping stone to seniority. However, the job is also suitable for a mature man who is happiest with his patients and lacks the desire or aptitude to become responsible for management. Our present assistant is 36 and a native of Ireland; he enjoys shooting and fishing in his spare time and is also master of the local masonic lodge. A sociable character, he is very popular with the patients and has made many friends within the village.

Whatever the age of the incumbent, this post is generally considered more appropriate for the single man, and most asylums do not provide married quarters for their assistant medics. The medical officer's accommodation here consists of a one-bedroom apartment above the patients' dining room. His salary is also slightly less than one quarter of the superintendent's, while his leave is a less generous four weeks. These restrictions make it difficult for such a gentleman to maintain a family home.

The medical officer's role is to support his superior physician. He does this by reporting anything of note or cases that require attention, and while he can suggest remedies, he may only act on them with permission from above. He does, however, maintain some day-to-day discipline amongst the attendants and acts as chief of the asylum during the superintendent's absence. To the medical officer also falls much of the patient care. His sole administrative responsibility is writing up observations into the asylum case books, thereby keeping a regular record of each patient's symptoms and health; otherwise, he is free to give himself up to ward rounds and study. He is always on hand to deal with daytime incidents, and can be summoned to deal with an emergency or medical crisis.

In practice, while the superintendent is asked to check on the sick or troubling cases, all the other wards are the province of his assistant for inspection on a daily basis. For this reason you can expect to see far more of the assistant officer than the superintendent. The nature of their shared responsibility is such that it is very rare to see both men attend the same ward at the same time, and each must rely on the other's information to gain a full picture of the institution.

As the principal practitioner of medicine within the asylum, it is the assistant's job to take charge of surgical equipment. He keeps our instruments dry and inspects them regularly for signs of damp or rust. If necessary, he sterilises them in a solution of potassium cyanide. These instruments are kept in the assistant's surgery room, though some items, such as tubes required for emergency or therapeutic procedures, are placed about the wards. The assistant also acts as apothecary and pharmacist. He manages supplies of drugs and spirits and keeps the dispensary stocked ordering supplies as required.

In most asylums the assistant officer is also tasked with some specialist jobs dependent on his skills. Increasingly an assistant is provided with a photographic studio, built against a north wall, in which he may take photographs of new admissions or patients ready for discharge. He is also expected to play a role in the sporting and artistic life of the asylum. Our present assistant is a most proficient musician, and will be found playing the piano at evening events and the harmonium each Sunday in chapel. He takes a leading role in dramatic entertainments and usually directs proceedings.

The Clerk and Steward

It is the steward's job to ensure the asylum is maintained and well supplied, and the clerk's to ensure that our paperwork is in order. In our small institution these two posts are combined, though in larger institutions the roles are separately demarcated. You may occasionally see our clerk and steward inspecting some part of the building. He is originally from Yorkshire, a Chelsea Pensioner and a family man.

As clerk, he is the head of our administrative staff, and under direction from the superintendent he keeps the books of record up-to-date, copying the details from admissions forms into various registers and transferring the lists of those departed into others. The clerk ensures that we conform to the requirements of record-keeping as set out by Parliament, and he sends notices and statistics to the Commissioners in Lunacy and the local poor law officers, also writing letters on the superintendent's behalf.

Our clerk is additionally tasked with the asylum's accounts, maintaining financial probity. In this he may be helped by a patient, if a suitably neat and accurate person can be found, or a former clerk who should require little direction or supervision.

In our asylum, the part of the job relating to the role of steward is by far the larger. For while the chaplain fulfils the spiritual needs of the patients, to the steward falls the material considerations of fabric, fittings, furnishings, food and fuel, clothing, sanitation, water, light and heat – the raw materials for each area must be ordered and then put to work. In some large asylums the steward is assisted by a storekeeper, but here he assumes ultimate responsibility for supplies, aided by the housekeeper on the female side. Our steward is below only the superintendent and chaplain in strict order of salary. He is also responsible for a number of servants who labour to create the comfortable conditions that surround you.

The steward is therefore a most practical man. He has an understanding of both commerce and construction. He must fathom the principles of drainage, imagine building alterations in his mind's eye, and predict the likely wear of cloths presented to him. These skills allow him to advise the superintendent, who is not expected to have such intimate knowledge of the world of manual labour.

The Housekeeper

The most senior female member of staff, the asylum housekeeper has significant responsibilities. To a certain extent she acts as a maternal superintendent on the women's side, combining her role with that of a head female attendant, and is tasked with the day-to-day management of that division. For this reason some asylums refer to the position as matron. The housekeeper's high standing is reflected in her terms and conditions: she is entitled to one months' leave per annum, which places her on the same level as the junior male officers, and also receives a salary slightly above that of the assistant medical officer.

Male patients are unlikely ever to see the housekeeper outside mealtimes or communal events, yet female patients look to the housekeeper, at least in the first instance, for all their needs. The housekeeper is directly responsible for the appearance of every patient in her care. It is her job to ensure the personal cleanliness of every female (particularly in regard to hands and hair), that their clothing is appropriate and neat, their bedding is fresh and that the wards and day-rooms on the female side are clean and free of dust. She does this through regular inspection, and as the superintendent and his assistant officer make their rounds to observe the patients' health, employment and intake of fresh air, so the housekeeper makes a similar round on the female side.

She takes at least two tours each day, usually in the morning, at mealtimes, or shortly before patients are put to bed. In the morning, she makes sure that everyone is out of bed and that the ward windows have been opened. She is present at the bathing of every female patient to check that the bath temperature is correct; at every mealtime to ensure that each patient takes her food; and to personally receive each new female admission. At night, she locks the communicating doors between the female side and the rest of the asylum, and she is also obliged to make occasional, unannounced nocturnal visits to the wards.

The housekeeper has in her charge all the female staff of the asylum, extending her jurisdiction beyond the wards and into the kitchen, the laundry, the sewing room and even the female attendants' personal quarters. All must be inspected and kept tidy, with each female attendant allocated a job according to a rota. This is a position of considerable power and should not be abused, though it is a well-known fact that women in authority are more susceptible to the influence of personal friendships or vendettas, and so the superintendent will maintain a regular interest in the housekeeper's supervision of her staff.

Nevertheless, it occasionally falls to the housekeeper to practise discipline. Attendants must be present for their duties, meals must be properly cooked and foodstuffs correctly stored, washing must be efficient and each garment sewn must be robust and comfortable to wear. In this regard it is helpful to have a separate stock of supplies to hand, and the housekeeper keeps a small store.

In some asylums, the feeling persists that the best housekeeper is a mature spinster who will not leave to be married and can thus provide continuity of care. Here, we have employed married women providing they are past the age of childbearing, as an experience of domesticity is invaluable in creating a home for so many people. However, we recognise that a married housekeeper is far more likely to fall prey to the pressures of asylum work; unless her husband is on the staff, the domestic home will be located some distance away from our main building. Our present housekeeper is a widow and therefore able to live in a flat on the premises.

The Asylum Attendants

The Head Attendant

Within the attendant class it has been found desirable to institute a level of supervision. In very large asylums this can be threefold, with a head attendant above those in charge of each annexe or block, and further charge attendants for each ward. Our asylum dispenses with the middle layer; but the post of head attendant is still required. A good head attendant holds a deep attachment to nursing and can give an equal priority to the circumstances of both his patients and his staff. He can lead by example and discipline those who do not follow his lead. He is obsessed with details of presentation, but not to the extent that he cannot see the wood for the trees. The values of an asylum can often be measured from the man who fills this role.

Our head attendant is a navy pensioner who grew up in the East End of London. He is married with three children, and has successfully studied for the certificate in proficiency available from the Medico-Psychological Association, which means that he is well-versed in the experiences of life as well as theoretical study of disorders of the mind and the care of the insane. To this theoretical knowledge he has added a period of work at an asylum 100 miles distant, so he is accustomed to the nature of this type of institution and the variety of patients found within it.

On the male side, the head attendant fulfils a more limited portion of the duties ascribed to the housekeeper, and so he is paid a remuneration of around half that of the senior female officer. His duties are no less significant, however, and he must construct the male staff duty rotas, ensuring that each attendant knows his daily role, and act as a conduit between his staff and the medical officers. The standard of cleanliness of the male patients, their clothes, bedding and wards is laid at his door. Like the housekeeper, he is also present at the reception and discharge of his patients.

Although he has his own office and an apartment on the ground floor of the main block, he is more usually to be found on duty within the wards, workshops or airing courts. He has the same responsibility for regular inspection as the housekeeper. Every morning he sees that each male patient is roused and that the windows have been opened, attends when bathing is in progress, is present at every meal to ensure that all are served, and also attends chapel, sporting events and entertainments to deploy his staff. He is expected to accompany the superintendent on the latter's rounds. The result is that in the men's wards you will see our head attendant regularly as the constant face of management, glimpsed briefly but consistently throughout each day.

The Attendants

It may seem cursory to group these staff together, but although they are legion – at any one time around thirty-six are on our books, divided roughly in half between each side of the asylum – each attendant performs the same duties. By far the greater number – some fifteen men and fifteen women – are on duty during daylight hours, while three guard the dormitories on each side at night.

The attendants are responsible for nursing care and these are the members of staff with whom you will forge the closest bonds. You may never register a new servant; you may notice only obliquely a different officer; but a change of attendant will be deeply felt. For this reason we do everything we can to stem the traffic of staff to pastures new. Even within the asylum, we try not to move attendants around too much. As a patient you will value the sight of familiar faces on the ward, which in their own way bolster your routine. You may feel anxious if a stranger wakes you in the morning or prepares you for bed at night. We understand this.

Nevertheless, you must prepare yourself for a somewhat high turnover of the staff, as only around half our attendants could be described as long-serving, and a loss of one in four a year is not uncommon. Unfortunately, this is mainly due to the terms and conditions of their employment, which are sadly outside our control. Nurses and carers must be paid a rate that preserves the asylum hierarchy and, while the ratepayers may be content to see larger sums paid to senior men, they will not tolerate the same expenditure on those of lower birth and education.

It is true that the attendants often feel hard done by. They are the first on duty, yet the last to leave or take their meals – and cold dinners do not make a man embrace his work. A few among them resent the speed with which they are admonished when compared to the slower thank-you for all that has gone well during the day. They have little control over their own duties and are not encouraged to have independent thought. They are the worker ants, without whom the colony would not endure but whose contribution does not find ready testimony.

Over time, the role of attendant has been seen increasingly as a specialism in its own right. Providing care is a more complex skill than those who built the asylum first conceded. As a result, we have managed to introduce some small changes to the attendants' terms of employment. Although each working day still begins at 6am, on each alternate day attendants are permitted to stop work at 8.30pm, rather than 10pm. Once a week, they are able to leave their duties at 3.30pm for a free afternoon. The beer ration they previously enjoyed has been converted into a more flexible monetary allowance and we have also purchased a terrace of nine cottages nearby to let to those attendants who require married quarters. We provide food to the attendants on duty, while those on night shift have their heated room in which to sit and view the ward.

Long service is rewarded with either a little extra pay or additional leave. There are opportunities too for advancement, and when the more senior posts of charge attendants become vacant we try to promote existing staff. We also endeavour to do what we can to remove the burdens of institutional life. Every attendant is allowed to tend an allotment in the kitchen garden; there is a quarterly dance to relieve the monotony of their routine; and a sumptuous meal of roast goose at Christmas, with lemonade and a dance to follow. Attendants who become unwell are offered the use of a seaside home in which to convalesce.

Uniform is issued to all attendants: a dark blue suit for the men and a similarly-coloured dress for the women, both available in seasonally appropriate, heavier or lighter fabrics. The men wear a dark blue cap, the women white caps and a fetching white apron with feathered straps. Each attendant has three sets of clothes so that they can present a smart appearance at all times. The attendants' dress forms a part of their nursing care, as it gives them authority that all but the most disorientated patients can recognise. The charge and head attendants are marked out more clearly by the gold braid on their caps and jackets, if they are male, and by a coloured ribbon around their caps if female.

You will easily be able to identify our newest recruits as they work here for a month in their own clothes. They are young men and women, usually in their early twenties, who have often come to employment from adjacent counties or from London. They are obliged to sign a declaration that they will dedicate themselves to the recovery of the patients and to securing their comfort, welfare and safety, while they are also issued with a copy of the rules and regulations for the governance of this asylum. These items form the foundations of their work.

Much has been written about the greater ease with which female asylum attendants can be found in contrast to equivalent male recruits and there is some truth in that. A male attendant has often tried other lines of profession first, without success, suggesting that his general suitability for work might be questionable. A female attendant has probably undertaken duties within the family home or may have some experience of domestic service, but she will have identified asylum care as her professional goal and set out to achieve it. The *quid pro quo*, of course, is the greater risk of losing female staff. The women are just as likely to quit their post for money or position, but additionally they must leave our labour upon marriage, in order that they can dedicate themselves to the family home and the prospect of maternity.

Yet female attendants are so much cheaper to hire, and so less has been invested in each new wife lost to us. This investment is partly in time and partly in study. Training for attendants is a comparatively recent development, but now that it is available we have embraced it. Many new attendants arrive fresh from the field or the scullery, and once garnered they must be capable of quickly absorbing a little of the human condition. Each new recruit is sent through the Medico-Psychological Association certificate, and we have additionally endeavoured to offer this route to our more established staff. Gone are the days when an attendant was selected for employment purely on their physical presence, and then placed in the ward to learn only from the memory of his closest colleague and through the bitter difficulties of experience. The modern attendant must have a range of knowledge at his or her finger tips.

This knowledge is then tested fully over a period of six months' probation. During those months new attendants work around each ward in turn. This is a necessary exception to our usual rule of continuity, as it is vital that each apprentice has experience of the different types of mental disorder and how these manifest in patients. A journey round the wards at speed is the best way to achieve this, but the result is that if you welcome a probationer to your ward then try not to form a great attachment to them.

Once fully trained, the new attendant should be able to employ the kindness, patience and understanding imperative within the asylum regulations. The regulations cover much of the usual daily business relating to patients which touch upon clothing, cleanliness and supervision, as well as instructions to inform senior staff of any incident or of any patient movements.

The language in which the regulations are written should leave you in no doubt that our organisation aims to present an attitude of beneficence at all times. Alienists have long since recognised that any creature, no matter how sick in mind, may be adduced to co-operation through the gentle application of the asylum routine by persons who display a soothing nature. There are, of course, penalties laid down in statute for any staff who ill-treat or wilfully neglect a patient, but it is our aim to do somewhat better than simple competence.

You should never be made to feel worse by an attendant; it is their duty to respond appropriately to your condition. Not even the most extravagant delusions will be mocked, yet nor will they be deferred to or encouraged. Attendants must refrain from making personal comments or discussing the case of any patient in public hearing. Suicidal patients will never be allowed alone, epileptic patients will be escorted up and down stairs, and the melancholy will be in receipt of cheery conversation. The quiet patient should receive protection from the boisterous and vice versa, the frail or timid should be protected from those prone to excessive demonstrations of force or high volume utterances. If another patient intimidates you, or makes you anxious, then the attendants on the ward will be alive to this possibility and seek to protect you.

Attendants are obliged to be industrious, so that they set a good example for the patients. The day attendants rise early and are late to bed. They are encouraged to take part in the occupations, amusements and other entertainments offered to the patients, to be creative in their use of occupation, and to use any opportunity to engage a patient in some helpful task.

The other essential part of an attendant's character is the ability to observe patients and to draw inferences about their behaviour. For the attendant is the superintendent's eyes and ears on every asylum ward. Two are on duty in any ward at any time and they will notice if you are acting out of character, or if any change has been detected in the atmosphere of the room. They will make reports on accidents, outbursts, illness or refusal of food. They are under strict instructions never to leave any ward, day-room or bathing room unsupervised, nor any window or door dangerously open.

The management of danger forms the last notable feature of the attendant's role. At times they must take action for the patients' safety, and when such eventualities occur an attendant will be firm with you, restraining you as necessary. The attendants are also aware at all times of the possibility of weapons being acquired or fashioned by patients, as many household objects can become sources of attack. From time to time it may be necessary for an attendant to search you, so please comply with their request. Similarly, you may find certain articles are removed from your possession or your ward, and if you have need of something, then please ask the attendants whether it can be granted.

Although the list of attendants' tasks seems daunting, you should think of them as the people whose primary task is to make your life comfortable and ensure you do not go hungry, dirty or unoccupied. A good attendant can address all things without the patients becoming aware that work is done.

Outdoor Servants

The Engineer

Every modern asylum needs a man who can understand the workings of heating and lighting apparatus. The boilers, engines and pipe work that deliver these marvels for our comfort all must be managed and maintained. The engineer performs this vital task, and the importance of his position is reflected in the wages offered to him - slightly higher than those of our head attendant - and the fact that he is also offered accommodation on the site. Emergencies are wont to occur at any time, such as when water froze around our gasometer one winter's night, impeding our supply, and it makes sense to have the engineer on immediate hand for their efficient rectification.

The engineer also acts as an inspector, checking the fuel systems and those of the asylum sanitation. If he finds that repairs are required, he will inform the steward of their cost and importance, so that his senior officer might decide a course of action. He oversees other essential jobs of housekeeping, ensuring that the chimneys are swept and the gutters cleared. You may occasionally see him deep in conversation with another member of staff, but he will not come and speak to you, nor should he, as his job places him behind the scenes.

The engineer additionally has a role to play in managing supplies. For he acts as a safety valve against excessive consumption, monitoring the use of gas, wood and coal by every ward. Irregularities are always investigated.

The Bailiff

As the engineer is to fuel, so the bailiff is to food. He manages our farm, our fields and gardens: if new spades are required, he will tell the steward; if we must purchase lambs, or pigs, or cows then he will identify the need and inform the visitors; when the time comes to order seeds he will construct the inventory. He also keeps a record of the dairy, eggs and crops that accrue to us. The bailiff is, therefore, another of our practical men, and you may never see him unless the farm is your place of work, but behind the scenes his keen understanding of nature, animals and the seasons is vital, and he puts it to good use. He also has a creative side: for it is under his direction that the planting of trees, shrubs or other plants is undertaken in the airing courts and gardens.

Asylum bailiffs have usually managed farms on country estates, and as you might expect, this means that they tend to be married men, which can provide additional benefits to the asylum. The wife of our present bailiff, for example, is engaged as our dairywoman and oversees the milking of the cows.

Other Outdoor Servants

The steward, the engineer and the bailiff obviously do not act alone. At any time, the operation of the asylum estate may have need of further help, and on the permanent staff we employ a gasman, whose sole responsibility is to oversee that element; a baker, whose task is to keep stocks of fresh bread plentiful; and a stoker, who loads the boilers. All these jobs must be filled by reliable persons who are careful and diligent. The roles of gasman and baker are considered so important for the running of the asylum that their salaries are comparable with that of the head attendant.

The bailiff also has the assistance of a permanent gardener, a man who can undertake the practical work of planting, directing a patient cohort to assist him. Then there is the carter, who transports supplies, as well as staff and patients, and collects further goods from local businesses. You will see him and his horses from time to time along the drive or hear the distant noise of hooves against the highway stones.

Additionally, we make use of a small number of seasonal labourers, who arrive at harvest time or to help with the regular maintenance of the building. They are paid higher wages in the summer, and a winter retainer to ensure they will return the following year. Bricklayers, painters and carpenters may all sometimes be seen about the estate and you could find yourself working with them, if you assist with labouring duties.

Indoor Servants

The indoor servants will be invisible to you, unless you are assigned to work at one of their stations. The three most senior indoor servants are the porter, the cook and the laundress.

The porter transports items from one place in the asylum to another, including foodstuffs, clothing and furniture. He works under the direction of the steward and provides a little assistance in the keeping of the stores. It is his responsibility to guarantee that no illicit liquors are brought into the asylum, and that no asylum property finds its way out. The cook is in charge of the running of the kitchens, and makes sure that food is readied and served for every meal, as well as keeping an eye on the larder stores for condition and for quantity. The laundress oversees wash days, drying, ironing and then the movement of clothes back into the stores. All three of these positions are paid at a higher rate than the attendants, and all three have extra junior staff to assist them.

These last posts must be considered at the bottom of our hierarchy: the gatekeeper (who logs the comings and goings of staff, as well as deliverymen); the kitchen maid, house maid; and two laundry maids. They have live-in accommodation provided, but at a salary around one twenty-fifth that of the superintendent's you may not be surprised to hear that they are usually filled by younger staff, who do not have the expense of a family.

Finally, we have a number of mechanic attendants who are not salaried employees, but are paid an hourly rate. These artisans look after the workshops: a carpenter, shoemaker, tailor and upholsterer. They are all expected to be off the asylum premises by 5.30pm after the shops have been closed for the day, the tools counted and the surfaces cleaned.

Staff Discipline

It is perhaps appropriate, before leaving the matter of staffing, to make reference to the question of discipline. The behaviour of staff is taken very seriously within the asylum. The superintendent has the power to summarily dismiss any of his staff, though a right of appeal exists to the committee of visitors. However, any member of staff wishing to challenge the superintendent's opinion will place the visitors in a difficult position, and it is extremely unlikely that they should wish to overturn their representative's judgement.

As in any institution the best discipline is often that which is administered immediately. Senior staff are encouraged to admonish any practice found wanting the instant it is discovered. Many such incidents require no further hearing or investigation and will never be set down in written form. To prevent any deterioration in performance, regular reports on attendants are received by the charge staff responsible for each ward. These will include notes of any occasion where staff have not met our high standards. Any complaint you might make against a member of staff will be included in such a report and ill discipline amongst the staff will be recorded. We keep defaulters' books, which act as the record of misdemeanours committed by the staff, and these include a note about subsequent enquiries and any action taken.

Most offences amongst the staff require no more than a warning. Attendants found sleeping on night duty by a senior colleague; who cannot account for a wandering patient or left a kitchen knife unattended; the man whose liquor-scented breath is discovered quickly upon his first "Good evening"; all these people are likely at most to have a note made against their name. Due to the nature of their tasks, it is the attendants who bear the brunt of such scolding. Nevertheless, they are not alone. One New Year's Day the porter failed to return to his post, having been sent the previous day to the nearest town to get change for a five pound note. He claimed that he could remember nothing between entering one of the borough's inns the night before and then waking up on board a train to London.

More serious offences might be dealt with by suspension; these are cases where behaviour has been exhibited that is wholly unacceptable. Staff are expected to behave in a proper manner at all times, and not to engage in base activity, including the use of indecent language in the servants' mess or other communal rooms, or harassment of the female staff. Another porter once employed would put nuts down the dresses of the younger staff and then try to retrieve them. A period of time without wages was felt to be a suitable response to his flagrant, indecorous conduct.

The ultimate sanction for misconduct is dismissal. Offences that lead to a summary parting of the ways are those that indicate a complete unsuitability for continued employment: an obvious or wilful neglect of duty, persistent drunkenness, a fraud or deception, or steadfast insubordination in relation to a senior colleague. Over recent years, two attendants have been dismissed following a fight between them; similarly, a proven assault upon a patient was enough to terminate the employment of another.

With transgressions of a moral nature such as these, an individual can usually be persuaded to do the honourable thing and resign. A male attendant who was intimate with a female colleague, resulting in her pregnancy, realised for example that it would be expedient for him to leave. The man who escorted his colleague's wife home from the railway station – and not by the most direct route available – also recognised that continuation of his employment would be undesirable.

Chapter 6

The Daily Routine

After your symptoms have been assessed, it is time to move you to whichever ward is most appropriate for your condition. This seems a suitable point at which to discuss your daily routine here. Routine is of the utmost importance to the asylum and its patients, as it allows for the asylum staff to know their stations, and for patients to understand the gentle forces applied to keep them active in the day.

To a certain extent, your daily routine is also determined by your symptoms. Some patients will be better able to partake of the wide range of activities we offer than others. Please accept this and do not struggle against it; the medical officers will take charge of what is suitable for you and they will instruct the attendants accordingly. Within these boundaries it is possible still to illuminate the features of an average day.

At the early, and consequently healthy, hour of 6am the day attendants come on duty (one hour later during winter), and this changeover from the night staff is the signal for all patients to rise. You will be wakened in good time to perform the necessary ablutions and evacuations. Convalescent patients in single rooms will be obliged to empty their chamber pots, while a similar activity is undertaken by the attendants in the dormitories. Those patients who have soiled themselves at night will be taken off to bathe.

Also in the dormitories the lavatory table will be procured for those able to wash themselves, and flannels provided for the purpose, while in the more secure wards the attendants apply the flannels to patients directly. Each patient's hair is combed and, if necessary, fixed-up for the day, and patients with false dentures are able to reclaim them. Patients with their own teeth will be allowed a toothbrush if they are capable of appreciating its use. Then it is time for all to change from their nightdress into daytime attire.

While you prepare for your day, the kitchen staff are busy with your breakfast. When everyone within the dormitory is ready, your ward attendants will direct you to file, in as orderly a fashion as you can muster, out of your dormitory and down the stone stairs. You wait in the lobby on your side of the central corridor and from there progress towards the benches and tables in the dining hall.

Breakfast begins at around 7am, or one hour later in the depths of winter. When all are present, grace is spoken. On the table before you the same fare is provided daily: an 8oz ration per patient of bread from the previous day's baking, cut into slices and coated with butter. This bread is mostly of brown whole-wheat or occasionally black rye. A tin mug sits waiting to be filled with tea from a pot as the attendants and their patient helpers make their rounds, and coffee is occasionally made available if it can be procured at an acceptable price.

Eating is a social experience but is also constrained by the clock. Like you, the staff have a routine and, unless you are in the infirmary ward, it will not be possible for you to prolong your breakfast beyond that of the other members of your ward. You are perfectly at liberty to talk but please be aware of the passage of time and that, inevitably, the moment must come when you have to put down your mug and leave the plate behind you, in order that the daily routine continues.

After breakfast some patients – around two in every ten – choose to attend chapel to hear the chaplain read the morning prayers. These begin at 8.20am, late enough that the sun will have risen on even the shortest winter's day. There is no requirement to attend religious service; indeed, in some patients there is a danger that it may induce or contribute to religious mania. We recognise also the practical difficulties of encouraging large numbers of patients to and from the chapel. As a result, attendance is largely restricted to those convalescent patients called by faith, who choose to proceed quietly to our place of worship in fine weather or foul.

Work and Occupation

After these first appointments of the day it is time to move on to work and occupation. This is not just a way of spending time but a vital part of your treatment here. Your improvement is contingent upon your industry. Many patients complain that they should not have to work and they reason that, as their treatment is forced upon them, they are under no obligation to assist with the smooth running of their surroundings, which some wrongly see as captivity. They also argue that if they are to give their labour then some recompense should be provided, as would be the case with any private employer.

These objections are ones of principle. For the latter objection, we provide recompense where we can. Extra rations are available to the working patient in the form of lunch and an allowance of beer and a wider range of clothing. For the former, we suggest that any aggrieved patient consider the wider picture. Not working might indicate an inability to live independently outside the asylum. Any patient unable to live independently is unlikely to be considered suitable for discharge and by remaining idle your fate is most determinedly to stay here also.

However, under no circumstances will we insist that you work. Indeed, we recognise that due to the nature of their illness many patients are simply unable to function in a productive manner. At any one time we estimate that around a third of our patient group falls into this category. The practice of asylums in managing these patients varies considerably. If your case is such then we shall still endeavour to keep you occupied, as even the most demented patient here, unless catatonic and immobile, can most likely be induced towards some mechanical action.

At its most basic level, this action can be found through the creative use of the waste of asylum life. Thus, old newspapers can be shredded to make stuffing for the bedding of patients liable to wet or soil themselves; horse hair can be combed to fill pillows; rags can be torn into fuel for the boiler. These tasks are inoffensive, undemanding and require no special tools or supervision; they even make productive use of patients who tend to be destructive. At this asylum we consider such activities to be a welcome addition to the daily output.

Most work performed by patients is unskilled. This is an inevitable consequence of the associated supervision required of any patient who wishes to undertake skilled labour. But there is an abundance of tasks that, while not requiring any exceptional talent, are of the utmost importance in providing an uplifting and healthy environment. They begin inside with the rigorous routine of cleaning required on all the communal places. Upon each ward there is a team of patient cleaners engaged in the washing, scrubbing and polishing of all the fixtures and fittings.

Around fifty patients, men and women, form these teams. Walk along any part of the asylum in the morning and you will see patients with mops, brushes or cloths in hand. Simple scrubbing can be easily taught and is a job available to the vast majority of patients. In some asylums, a little vinegar in used in the water to clean the floors and windows, though here we prefer to use soft soap or soda, so that the rooms and corridors do not retain the lingering, rather burning, smell of vinegar. Even so, during and after cleaning all available windows will be left open to allow the evaporation of any disagreeable chemicals.

Furniture and woodwork may be polished using a little oil. And if a patient feels uncomfortable with a bucket at their feet, then they can always pick up a drying cloth and follow on behind the wet work. Rugs from the day-rooms are taken outside and beaten by patients capable of wielding a carpet beater.

Outside work is also a regular activity for the male patients. Another 50 men work daily in the farm or kitchen garden, while additional seasonal duties may be required if building work is in progress. Work in the farm or gardens follows the same patterns as for the labourer of rational mind. The preparation of the land, the nurturing and harvesting of grains, fruits and vegetables are practised here in traditional fashion. To work in the kitchen garden is to enjoy the trust of using forks, hoes and spades – tools that may not be considered safe in all patients' hands. There is an element also of independence, for, while the attendants will watch you, there is always such a variety of tasks in hand that it is impossible for their eyes to be fixed on every mixed border. If you are detailed for the kitchen garden, then we suggest you use your privilege wisely, as it is a step along the pathway to discharge.

Work to the lawns, trees and shrubs is equally vital. A small sum is available each year for planting of new shrubs or other perennials, and we constantly strive to make the gardens a pleasing environment in which patients can recuperate. During the spring and summer months, the grass is kept neat by a team who use the cutting machines and a roller for ground levelling or maintaining the cricket pitch. The use of these tools is another privilege, especially in the less secure gardens to the front of the estate, while those teams who trim the specimen plants and boundary hedging with shears or loppers are also trusted, if rigorously supervised.

A careful eye is placed too upon those patients who help with the livestock on the farm. Inevitably, the farm bailiff has call only for a handful of workers, and these men must be amongst the most gentle of our patient group. If chosen, you may find yourself shepherding creatures to graze or to milk, or providing a comfortable environment for the pigs, sheep, cows and chickens through clearing old straw or laying fresh. There are daily tasks for the kitchen too, with butter to be churned and eggs to be retrieved from the coops and delivered to the larders.

Field work is more likely to be undertaken by patients in a small group, working together on a set task of digging, spreading manure, sowing or reaping. We employ seasonal labourers to thresh and undertake more dangerous activities, but there are still many opportunities for patients to help. Wheat, barley and oats are all tended on our wider estate and contribute to the bread we bake and the hot meals we provide, with any excess being sold; a significant quantity of potatoes are also grown to augment the grains in broths and stews.

At harvest time, you will find a swell in the numbers of patients directed to help in the fields and gather in the crops. There is a sense of community in this work, perhaps as great as you would find in any country parish. The same small group approach is true for the labours of building maintenance or building improvements. All the walkways and pathways around the airing courts, for example, were dug and laid to gravel with a coal tar surface by the patients. Other patients worked to extend these tarred tracks across the whole estate. The grounds between the main building and the river have been terraced, allowing for their better cultivation; the site for the asylum sewage works was levelled; stones have been broken to help provide foundations for building works; and hard landscaping – including a little brickwork – has been provided around some of the buildings. Recently a small group also undertook the arduous and unpleasant task of draining the cess pit.

Routine decoration is something you might help with, if you have the requisite neatness required for painting. Because of the accumulated effects of burning the stoves and the gas lamps, each year we try to whitewash the ceilings throughout the entire main building. Usually, at least one of the male or female sides is also repainted with the appropriate colour wash, while a smaller programme attempts to refresh the exterior wood and metalwork. That is recoated with an oil-based paint within a period of three to four years.

The same limitations are true of assisting in the workshops, which is perhaps the most exacting work that we can offer. Every good asylum is able to supply and look after its own clothing and fixtures, and we take pride in our own output. As a result, those patients with sufficient dexterity may find themselves invited to take up employment with one of our artisan attendants.

Our capacity is such that around twenty working men might join our permanent artisans – the shoemaker, tailor, upholsterer and carpenter – while one or two more might be invited to help the baker or the engineer, or assist the farrier should he visit. The workshops are equipped with stools and benches at comfortable heights, with trays of instruments always to be returned to their homes. In the shoemakers' shop there is the strong, sweet smell of leather, untempered by the usual odours of a tanner's shop, while cloth and wood bring a fresh aroma to the other workrooms.

Aside from cleaning, we prefer that female patients perform indoor work and they can bring their domestic skills to bear in three sections of the asylum: the laundry, the sewing room, and, to a lesser extent, the kitchens. As you may surmise, only our convalescent women are trusted with a needle. Within their pretty day-room, the casual visitor will happen upon a group of ladies, tastefully attired and engaged in needlework, as one might see in a domestic drawing room.

Altogether, we have space to accommodate around thirty seamstresses in the sewing room. It is like a small cottage industry, interrupted only by the healthy conversation of improving minds. Of course, much of the work comprises basic necessities: repairs to asylum garments, bed linen or washing materials. The women's own garments are also made here, but the cloth is first cut by an attendant and then sewn under her direction into patterns. The women patients who sew are also encouraged to work on their own items of clothing, as the crocheting of lace trimmings for a dress can help boost feminine esteem, as can the sewing of a dress with gay pattern from a non-standard cloth. These dresses can be made for themselves or for their patient friends, assuming such a gift is also beneficial to the other patients' health.

Laundry work is rather different, as it is far more oppressive to the senses. When the laundry is in operation there is much noise from both the hand and mechanised washing, the powerful (though not unpleasant) smell of tar from the carbolic soap, as well as a great heat and humidity created by the ironing and the drying cabinets. You will also deduce that wet clothes gain weight in excess of their dry poundage, and so a suitable candidate for the laundry will be of a robust nature, with physical strength and stamina, rather than one of our more delicate females. Nevertheless, we must always endeavour to find some thirty candidates so that we can rotate their duties, and also on occasions dispense with the need for the machines.

The laborious nature of washing, rinsing and drying so many clothes means that it is not possible for the laundry to be in operation every day. Washing occurs on three days of the week, with the fallow periods allowing for the clothes to be aired, collected and returned to store, ready for the rotation of the patients' linen. Thus, if you work in the laundry, you will find that your work has a routine varying between wet days and dry days.

Finally, a small number of our female patients help in the kitchen. Kitchen work carries many risks, as there is a constant need for boiling water and feeding the fire in the stoves, as well as ready access to a surfeit of knives and other tools that can cause much harm in the wrong hands. In consequence, female help here is best used in the scullery, where plates, dishes and cutlery are washed and stored, or in the dining hall as servers; only the most trusted patient may assist with the preparation of food.

For Those Who Cannot Work, or for Working Patients in Possession of Some Idle Time

An asylum is a unique public institution in that the recreation of the patients is of as great importance as their work or custody. Those unable to enjoy the fruits of performing labour still join with the workers to engage in activities which do not necessarily have a purpose other than to stimulate and occupy. That is not to say that recreation is aimless, but rather that it need not lead to any immediate, visible product. As recreation is both healthy and good for the treatment of patients, we encourage it, and provide a wide range of amusements for all to enjoy.

Fresh Air Recreations

Let us begin with a simple perambulation in the enclosed airing courts, where paths frame the lawns and seats. Walks within the airing courts are suitable even for the infirm or for those at risk of becoming excitable. There is also a wider series of pleasant strolls available via the walkways around the estate. Of course, the necessary strength and behaviour to complete the walk is required, but around two-thirds of our patients take advantage of this latter option. Daily you will see groups of four or five taking the air along the river meadows or through the fields, each group accompanied by an attendant. Male and female groups always walk in opposite directions so that they do not meet.

Recently, we have been able to extend the scope of the walking parties to some of the lanes bordering the asylum and even the main road outside the gates, as it is infrequently traversed by carts and carriages. The female patients also enjoy these routes, as modern society no longer considers it quite so shocking to see a group of women walking, unaccompanied by a male chaperone, along the public roads.

For those patients who are unable to move beyond their wards, some assistance is given so that they may exercise through physical support or even a repetitive stretching and relaxing of the muscles. No patient is permitted to spend his or her time entirely at rest in the day-room or the ward corridor, lest this inactivity become a disagreeable habit.

More complex outdoor amusements tend to be the preserve of summer months. For the men, a cricket pitch was laid out in our inaugural summer, a year that also saw the asylum's first victory over the local village team. In due course we were able to create a permanent pitch complete with its own small pavilion, where patients may change their clothes in comfort. Now that the game of cricket has also been codified by the Marylebone Club, regulation equipment is quite easy to procure and cricket is played on every fine evening in the warmer seasons.

Umpires and scorers are found from amongst the convalescents, while the boundary line is replete with those too frail to participate, but who live out each triumph and disaster as if it were their own. To see cricket played as the sun gently slips beneath the summer sky, and a golden evening turns copper pink, is a true pleasure and no better picture of a harmonious assembly might be witnessed in any English village.

We act as hosts for cricket games against various local teams – including the asylums nearest to us – and are occasionally able to play return fixtures. The staff, of course, join in too, and each team has a mix of staff and patients. The patients enjoy the equal status that sport gives them with their warders and matches are keenly fought. One patient, who suffers from delusions of grandeur, is determined to maintain his status as the best bowler here (if not in the world), while our poor chaplain was struck by the ball during one innings last July and then was absent for several days.

In the winter months, we have found that the men enjoy the somewhat rougher pursuit of association football. Asylum football has its own rules, which consider excessive physical contact a disagreeable element to the game. Patients are therefore encouraged to play the ball and to leave the other players well alone, lest collision proves an unfortunate provocation to violence. It is for this reason that the rugby style of football is never practised in asylums.

While the women do not engage in team sports, the provision of a lawn tennis court has been of considerable benefit to them. We have a level site and it is a simple matter each year to mark out the lines of a court with twine and pegs, before painting them; a basic net of wooden posts and wire mesh lasts the season. As one might expect, there is less interest in sport on the female side, and it is easy to accommodate all the ladies who wish to play – using doubles where necessary – and still avoid playing during the heat of the day.

A growing number of less rigorous games are also finding their way into asylum life. Outdoor croquet, for example, is most suited to the restrictions of an airing court and can be played by a number of convalescing patients in less hospitable weather than is required for cricket or for tennis. A set of lawn bowls has been purchased for more elderly residents, and the creation of a bowling area is under active consideration.

Recreations Enjoyed Indoors

While activities outdoors are, of necessity, determined by the weather, activities inside the wards are offered daily as a staple way to occupy the irrational mind when it is not at work. On the convalescent wards some of these activities are available for patients to undertake by themselves; on the acute or refractory wards, the offer is more restricted.

Reading is perhaps the most common pursuit and every ward receives a daily supply of newspapers and an occasional supply of periodicals, so that any patient with an interest in reading can keep up their habit. The appropriation of newspapers for individual use is considered unacceptable, and the attendants will make sure that the day's stock remains accessible to all. There is no censorship of news, nor have we found any evidence that the editorial rigour of certain publications causes distress to patients. Newspapers and magazines are happily also disposable, so that should an accident befall a copy it creates no unforeseen dent in the institution budget.

Each ward is additionally supplied with three standard texts: a Bible, prayer and hymn books. Other reading matter is available from the asylum library; this collection is kept secured, but can be open to any patient upon application to the chaplain. The chaplain uses his discretion over how the library is stocked, and he procures volumes of general literature with advice from the Society for Promoting Christian Knowledge, who also supply the books. Their preference is for light fiction with moral tales, or factual works on matters of natural, scientific or historical interest. This year we have added the *Waverley* novels of Sir Walter Scott and a collection of Lord Bulwer-Lytton's popular stories. Books are issued on a monthly basis and a strict record is kept of each volume loaned. Each ward also has a bookcase where volumes can be kept safely when not required.

The other principal ward activity is the playing of indoor games. Cards are freely available, because like newspapers they are innocuous and easy to replace. In wards where it is safe to do so, sets of draughts, dominoes, bagatelle boards and chess are provided, though these are locked away when not in use. They may be issued under the supervision of an attendant, who can also supply a copy of the rules of each game to prevent controversy. During inclement seasons we bring out an indoor croquet set, as games may be played within the ward corridors. Finally, after many years of saving, we have recently been able to purchase a billiard table for use in the entertainments hall.

Other Daily Activities

Dinner is served at 12.30pm, when the workers rejoin their less active fellows. As at breakfast, the sexes progress from their separate lobbies into the dining hall, then sit at table waiting to be served.

The principal diet at the asylum is designed to provide foods of a starchy, fatty nature. This provides the bulk and substance required for physical work. Around two-thirds of your sustenance is based around bread or potatoes, with the other third provided by other foodstuffs. Many animals can survive happily on a diet of starch and fat alone, but we recognise that your morale may be raised and your digestion eased if supplied with a little variety. The high proportion of bland starch is also designed not to over-excite patients, as meat or other proteins may. Generally speaking, the lunatic patient suffers from excess energy, and therefore foods rich in nutrients are best given in gentle doses.

Dinner is the meal that provokes the greatest enthusiasm among patients, because meat is served. This may be boiled or roasted mutton, beef or pork: last year, we consumed over 5,000lbs of beef and over 3,000lbs of mutton from the farm, while an additional 500lbs of pork was purchased by the bailiff. We make efficient use of this weight and are keen to ensure that no part of an animal is left unused. Once a week, the leftovers are turned into stock to make a nourishing soup. This is supplemented with barley or another grain.

Each week, assorted meat pies are also baked in the ovens, with the pastry allowing for a slight reduction in the bread ration for the day; while on Friday, an Irish stew is prepared from other trays of unused cuts. Saturday's midday meal supplies the sweetest treat of the week, when either a meat suet pudding or, in season, plum or another type of fruit pudding is cooked. There are also exceptional occasions when we purchase a catch of freshwater fish or are presented with a gift of birds or rabbits by one of the local landowners.

The dinner fare is served with boiled potatoes, cooked in their jackets, though a quantity will be peeled for patients who struggle to chew their food. Vegetables may also be provided, with cabbage by far the most common sight upon our tables, with seasonal root or sprouting vegetables furnished by our kitchen garden.

The farm and garden grant such luxuries to us throughout the year. Roughly every pound spent on procuring victuals is matched by one pound's worth of goods produced here. On their most recent visit, for example, the Commissioners in Lunacy dined on our own bacon and cabbage in addition to our supplier's cold beef. At harvest time the garden also yields various fruits, some of which are stored over winter or made into preserves. When the garden cannot provide, then currants and other dried fruits are purchased to allow some extra sweetness into the diet; while treacle, rice, eggs, butter and flour are mixed for puddings to be served on special occasions. Cheese, milk, salt, pepper and spices are all used to enhance the dishes. Whatever the daily menu, there is no want of flavour.

Each meal is prepared in the kitchen and then transferred to a wagon and taken to the benches by an attendant or helper. Portions generally come in a standard size; 8oz of bread or potatoes added to a similar quantity of the meat, soup or pudding is recommended by the regulations, unless a special diet is required. One of the attendants' tasks is to observe their charges and report any problems that are had with eating or digesting food, or any tendency to eat unsuitable items such as stones or coal. For those unable to digest bread, an oatmeal porridge or similar recipe can be made up.

A cloth is placed upon each table, bibs are available for those who need them, and every patient's meal is served onto a tin plate covered with enamel. Grace is said. Ale and beer are the principal drinks at dinner, though in dilute form. Beer is known to be a most wholesome and beneficial drink, and many among the labouring classes retain a very strong affection for it. There has been some debate amongst our committee about whether beer should be reserved solely for the workers, and these discussions continue. For those who do not like the taste of beer, the alternative accompaniment is cold milk. Water is not recommended, unless served as a hot drink with oatmeal added to it.

In addition to your plate and beaker, table knives and spoons are available to all, though forks are provided only to the convalescent patients. Human dignity must be balanced with security, as cutlery is a potential source of danger, and every piece must be accounted for. Please do not attempt to remove articles for your own use.

When dinner is complete, patients will return to their previous activities, meeting up once more between 5 and 6pm for the last meal of the day: tea - or supper, which consists of a further 8oz ration of bread and butter, together with a mug of tea. This is carried out so that every patient is sent to bed with a full stomach and having had a hot drink.

Unless there is an evening entertainment, the period after supper allows time for reflection on the achievements of the day and a chance to converse together or play quiet games before bed. At this time male workers are most likely to make use of their allowance of tobacco. Although some patients smoke a lit pipe – one left in a jacket pocket once nearly caused a fire in the clothes store – most chew a handful of the leaves before they spit the remnants into a bowl or bucket. The smell of tobacco across the wards is one of the features of the evenings here.

At 7.30pm, the attendants will signal the day's end by closing the window shutters in the day-rooms. Conversations may be interrupted, games brought to a close and readers asked to close their volumes of improving text. The stoves are secured, the lights turned out and the patients are escorted from each room. The day-rooms are then locked and the keys returned to the charge attendant, while each group of patients files away towards their sleeping quarters.

This seems an appropriate point at which to consider the matter of bathing. While it is true that bathing may be undertaken at any time of the day as a patient's needs require, during the evening time is deliberately set aside to enact each patient's weekly bath. Every ward has a rota for bathing and, as it is necessary to bathe several patients in one session, there is no time to idle in the porcelain tub. Rather, there is a strict focus on your personal cleanliness, and the whole operation is directed by your charge attendant, who will engage junior attendants to assist with the process.

On your bath day, you will be expected to strip down to your undergarments and then await your turn. In the bathroom, the charge attendant will see that the bath is properly prepared. Cold water is first run in a moderate quantity, before that tap is stemmed and hot water added. It is vital that this procedure is followed: when a poor, idiot boy jumped unbidden into hot water he was scalded badly, and the attendant in charge was immediately given his notice. The increasing heat of the bath is tested continuously by the immersion of a thermometer until the temperature arrives at the range of ninety to ninety-six degrees Fahrenheit.

At this point, the junior attendant will fetch a patient, complete their undress and then supervise them as they bathe. Bathing is performed to an established routine: the patient will be immersed first in the water, before being requested to stand. Carbolic soap is then liberally applied – by the staff if the patient is unable, or unwilling to oblige – and then a coarse brush is agitated against the flesh to release the dirt and allow the soap to work into the skin. The hair is also thoroughly wetted. The patient is then dipped into the water once more to rinse the soap off. When the patient leaves the bath the water is run out, as it is not hygienic for multiple patients to bathe in the same water.

On leaving the bath, the attendant will first sponge off excess water from you, which then enables the person to be more effectively dried with a towel. A comb to seek out vermin will be brushed through the hair; if any are found, you will have your hair washed promptly with an insecticide. Finger and toe nails are clipped and male patients may be shaved under the direction of an attendant. Razors are available only to those shortly to depart on trial, and always under the strictest supervision.

For female patients, an additional weekday night is allowed for hair-washing, a process which cannot be adequately concluded within the usual time allotted for bathing. Female patients may also have their wet hair cut by the attendants, while women who require sanitary materials will be pleased to note that clean rags are made available in the female stores.

With the exception of bathing, there is not the same frenzy of washing before bed as can be seen at first light. The portable wash basin in each ward can be brought out for those who wish to use it, while those patients who drool or are inclined to dirty their hands or faces will be sponged before they retire.

When all patients are in their nightdress you will notice that there are some additional staff. The day shift has ended, and it is now the turn of the night attendants to offer you their care. They will invite you to go to bed; the expectation is that all patients will be settled by 8pm. The shutters in the

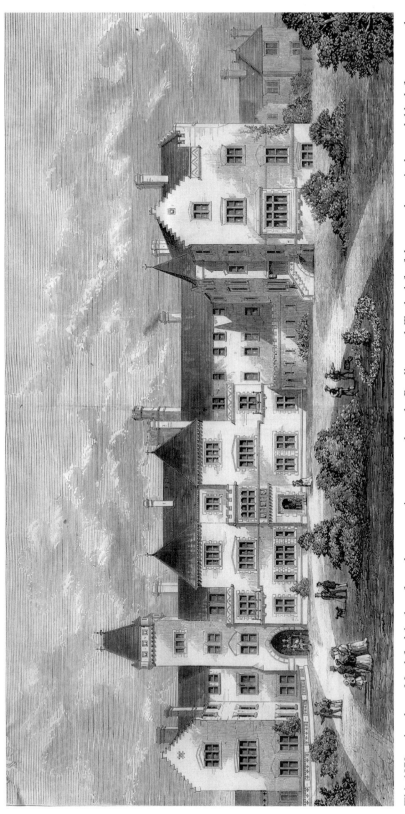

This 1870s print shows Moulsford Asylum from the west, at its entrance along the Reading road. To the left of the central core is the north block for men; to the far right is the superintendent's accommodation and between them, the north block for women. The women's south block can be seen in the background. *Reading Libraries.*

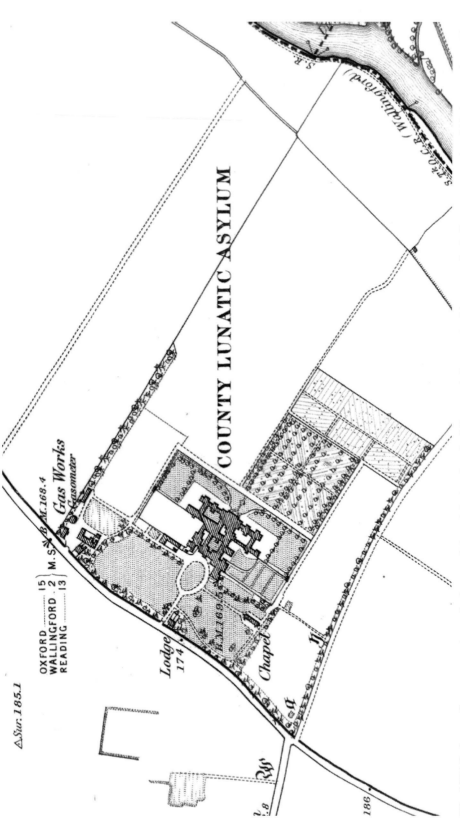

The 1877 Ordnance Survey map shows the layout of the original asylum buildings and the extent of its estate, including ornamental and kitchen gardens. The south blocks are those facing the river, while the north blocks face the road. The chapel is seen to the south west and the farm to the north of the principal buildings; the gas works are a little distant.

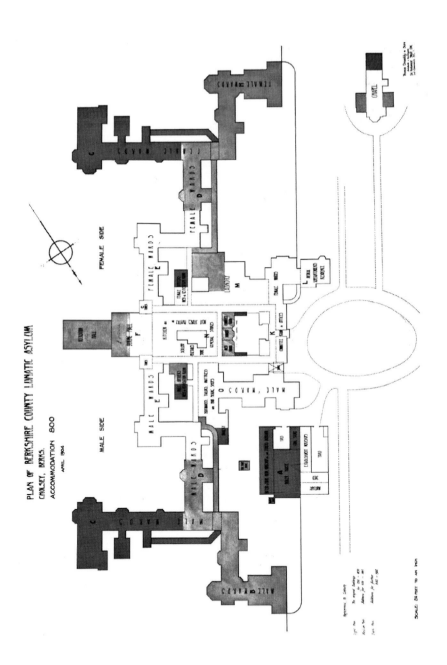

This 1904 surveyor's plan of Moulsford shows in more detail the different areas on the ground floor. The lightest shade also shows the buildings' original extent in 1870; the darker colours show the extensions made between then and the beginning of the twentieth century. *The Berkshire Record Office.*

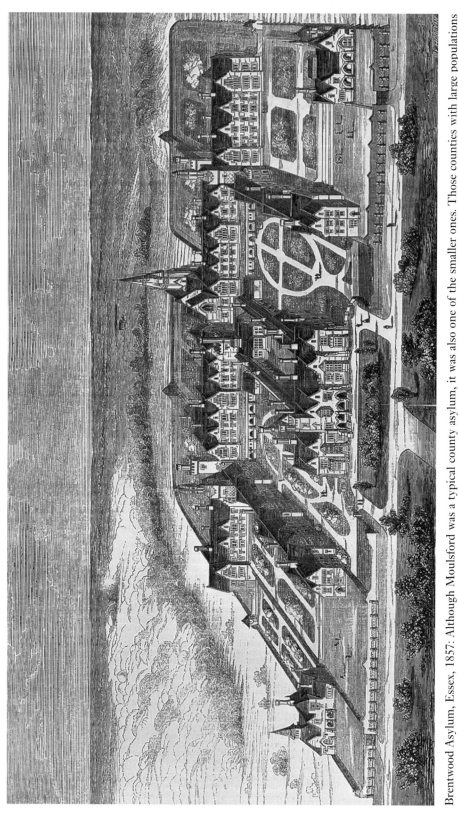

Brentwood Asylum, Essex, 1857: Although Moulsford was a typical county asylum, it was also one of the smaller ones. Those counties with large populations built on a grander scale. Here is the Brentwood Asylum, Essex, which opened in 1853 with beds for 450 patients. By the end of the century it had grown to accommodate 2,000 people. *Wellcome Library, London.*

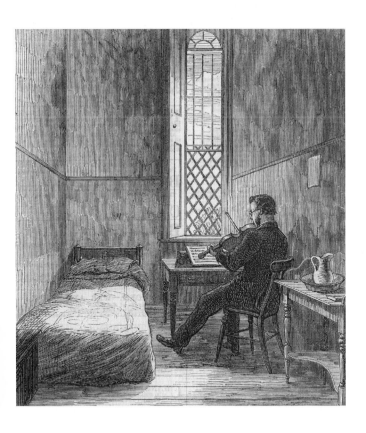

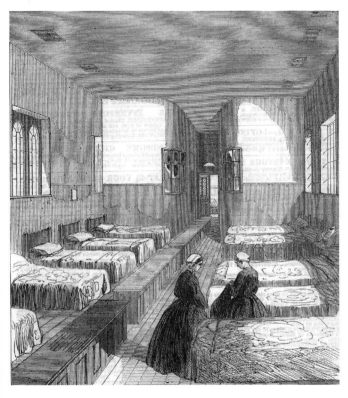

The patient sleeping spaces at Broadmoor: similar to those found elsewhere in the public system. Dormitories, in which by far the greater number of county pauper lunatics found themselves, contained neat rows of beds and storage for patients' night or day clothes. Single rooms might be used for patients at risk of harming others or, as here, approaching discharge. *Reading Libraries.*

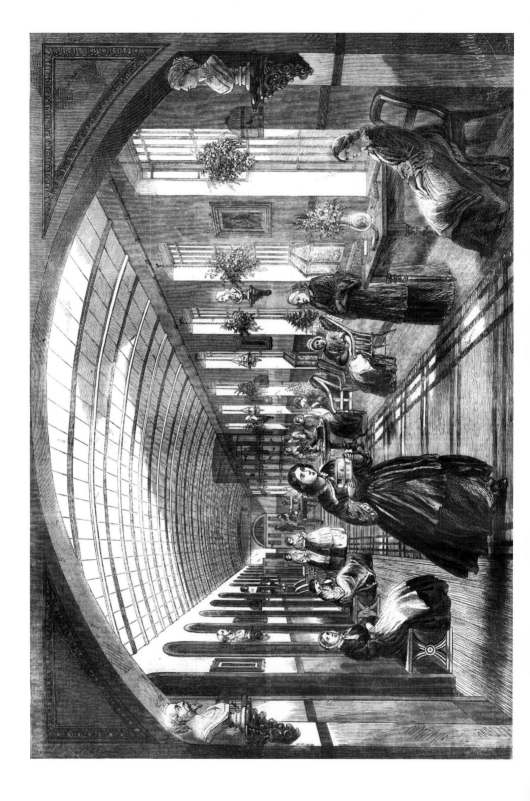

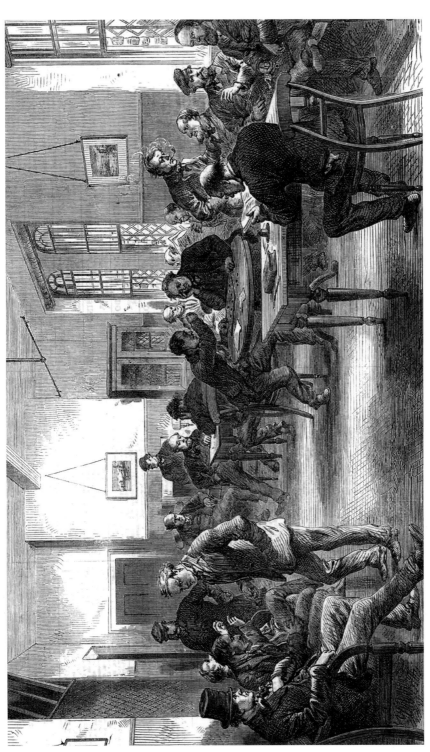

Two images from the *Illustrated London News* depict convalescent spaces at the Royal Bethlem Hospital and Broadmoor respectively. The scene in the Broadmoor dayroom, drawn in 1867, was replicated throughout the public asylums of England and Wales. Patients talk, sit, read or play games in a sparsely furnished but light and airy room. The women's gallery at Bethlem – including various caged birds – was drawn in 1869. Its décor is slightly grander than that of a public asylum. *Reading Libraries.*

TABLE X.

Showing the probable Causes, Apparent or Assigned, of the Disorder, in the Admissions, Discharges, and Deaths of the Year 1875.

CAUSES.	The Admissions.			The Discharges. Recovered.			Removed, Relieved, or otherwise.			The Deaths.		
	Males.	Females.	Total.	Males.	Females.	Total.	Males.	Females.	Total.	Males.	Females.	Total.
MORAL:												
Fright	...	1	1	...	...	...	...	...	...	...	...	...
Loss of Situation	1	...	1	...	...	...	...	...	...	...	...	...
„ Income	...	...	...	...	...	...	...	...	...	1	...	1
Religious Excitement	...	1	1	...	1	1	...	...	...	...	...	...
Suicide of Father	...	...	...	...	1	1	...	...	...	...	...	...
PHYSICAL:												
Amenorrhœa	...	1	1	...	1	1	...	...	...	...	...	...
Brain Disease	2	...	2	...	...	...	...	...	...	1	...	1
Chorea	...	...	...	...	...	...	1	1	2	1	...	1
Concussion of Brain	1	...	1	...	...	...	...	...	...	...	...	...
Congenital	1	1	2	...	...	...	...	...	...	...	1	1
Epilepsy	1	3	4	...	...	...	1	...	1	...	...	...
Hereditary	5	13	18	1	5	6	1	1	2	3	2	5
Hyperlactation	...	1	1	...	2	2	...	...	...	...	...	...
Injury to Head	2	...	2	...	...	...	...	...	...	2	...	2
Intemperance	5	...	5	4	1	5	...	1	1	1	...	1
Liver Disease	...	1	1	...	...	...	...	...	...	...	...	...
Menorrhagia	...	1	1	...	1	1	...	...	...	...	...	...
Old Age	...	1	1	...	...	...	...	...	...	...	...	...
Paralysis	...	...	...	...	...	...	...	...	...	...	1	1
Predisposition from Previous Attack	3	2	5	1	...	1	...	...	...	...	1	1
Puerperal State	...	3	3	...	1	1	...	...	...	...	...	...
Sun-stroke	1	...	1	...	...	...	...	...	...	1	...	1
Unascertained	10	10	20	2	3	5	...	4	4	8	6	14
Total	32	39	71	8	16	24	3	7	10	18	11	29

This page from Moulsford's annual report of 1875 shows superintendent Robert Gilland's attempts to assign a cause for each of his patients' illnesses. Just under a third of cases in this year were assigned no obvious trigger; in a further quarter only a vague attribution to 'hereditary' factors was made. *The Berkshire Record Office.*

TABLE No. 3.

Showing the Occupation or Station in Life of the Patients admitted in 1880.

Males.	Total.	Females.	Total.
Assistant Gamekeeper...	1	Bonnet Maker	1
Blacksmith	2	Cabman's Daughter ...	1
Brass Moulder	1	Carpenter's Widow	1
Bricklayer	1	Carpenter's Wife ...	3
Brickmaker	2	Charwoman	1
Carpenter	2	Companion to a Lady...	1
Carrier's Agent... ...	1	Divorced Wife of a Clerk	1
Carter	1	Domestic Servant ...	19
Clerk	3	Dressmaker	1
Draper	1	Farmer's Daughter ...	4
Factory Labourer ...	1	Field Labourer	6
Farm Labourer... ...	7	Gardener's Wife ...	1
Gardener	2	Governess	3
Groom	1	Groom's Wife	1
Harness Maker ...	2	Harness Maker's Widow	1
Innkeeper	1	Hawker	1
Labourer	24	Housewife	9
Painter	2	Labourer's Widow ...	2
Plumber	1	Labourer's Wife ...	13
Postman...	1	Mangle Woman ...	1
Printer	1	Patient's Wife	1
Railway Guard	1	Pauper	2
Ropemaker	1	Publican's Wife ...	1
Schoolmaster	1	Railway Porter's Wife...	1
Shoemaker	2	Sempstress	1
Shop Porter	3	Smith's Widow	1
Soldier	1	Tailor's Wife	1
Steward in the Navy ...	1	Tramp	1
Stonemason	1	Upholsterer's Widow ...	1
Tobacconist	1	Washerwoman	1
Occupation Unknown ..	2	Wheelwright's Wife ...	1
Of no Occupation ...	17	Occupation Unknown ...	7
		Of no Occupation ...	15
Total	89	Total	105

A table from the annual report of 1880 shows the wide range of occupations within just one year's worth of admissions to Moulsford. Although by far the greater number of new patients were either labourers or their wives, middle class Victorian life was also represented. Note also the increase in the number of annual admissions from the annual report of five years earlier. *The Berkshire Record Office.*

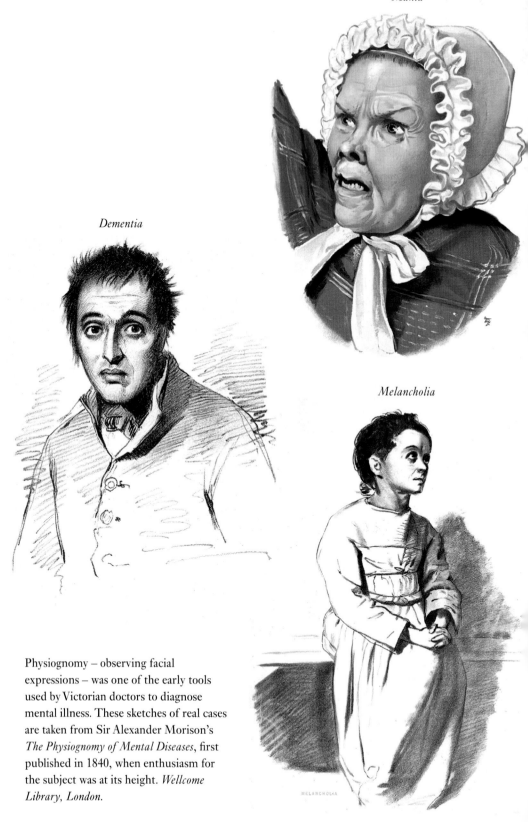

Mania

Dementia

Melancholia

Physiognomy – observing facial expressions – was one of the early tools used by Victorian doctors to diagnose mental illness. These sketches of real cases are taken from Sir Alexander Morison's *The Physiognomy of Mental Diseases*, first published in 1840, when enthusiasm for the subject was at its height. *Wellcome Library, London.*

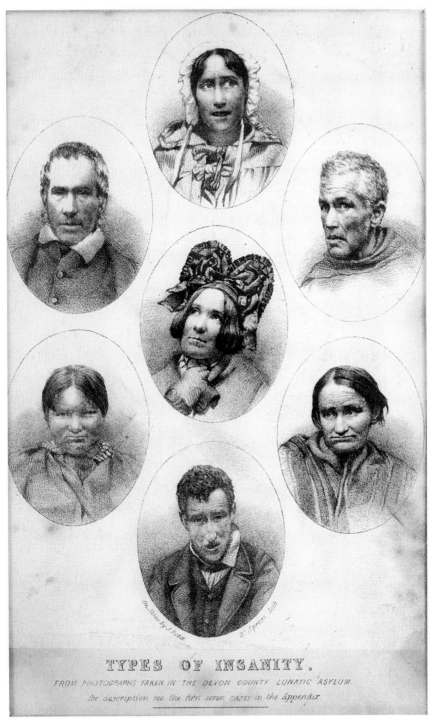

TYPES OF INSANITY.

FROM PHOTOGRAPHS TAKEN IN THE DEVON COUNTY LUNATIC ASYLUM.

for description see the first seven cases in the Appendix

Sketches of patients in the Devon Asylum. Clockwise from top: mania caused by destitution in a young mother; an older man with acute melancholy; a demented patient suffering hallucinations of a past lover; a 27-year-old man described as a 'congenital imbecile'; a 40-year-old woman with dementia; a middle-aged man with general paralysis. In the centre, the daughter of a customs officer, afflicted with monomania and convinced she was Queen Victoria. *Wellcome Library, London.*

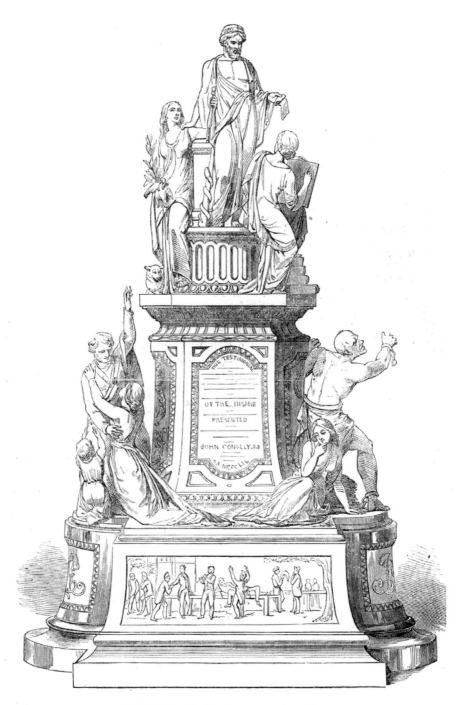

TESTIMONIAL PRESENTED TO DR. CONOLLY.

John Conolly, first resident physician at the Hanwell Asylum, was very influential. He established the moral regime in public institutions and was one of the first to dispense with restraint and show that a humane approach could work. When he retired in 1852, Conolly was presented with this 'testimonial'. The figures on its right depict mania and melancholia, while on the left those same figures are recovered. *Reading Libraries*.

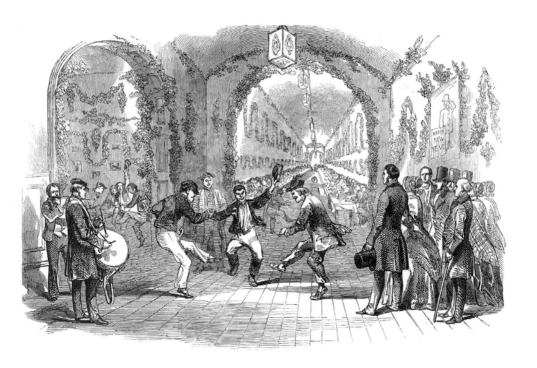

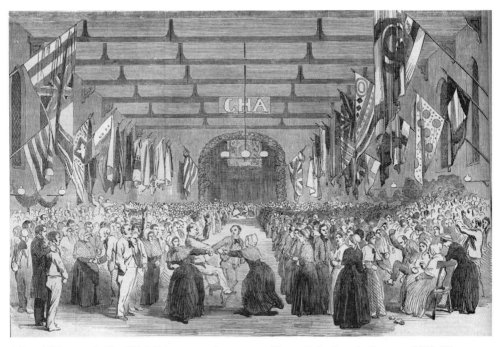

(*Above*) The men's Twelfth Night entertainments at Hanwell Asylum in January 1848. There was singing and dancing from 4.30pm until 8.00pm, when a supper of roast beef and vegetables was served with beer. (*Below*) Here the sexes are mixed for festivities at Colney Hatch on 4 January 1853. The officers staged a play, there were sung solos by selected patients, and finally the attendants and servants performed an 'Ethiopian dance'. *Reading Libraries.*

THEATRE 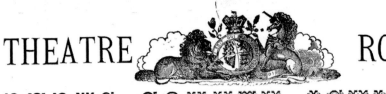 ROYAL,

BERKS COUNTY ASYLUM,

THURSDAY, NOVEMBER 15th, 1877.

It is with much pleasure that the Manager of this well-known Theatre announces, that he has, after a severe struggle with the Proprietor, in which he received a black eye and a broken nose, succeeded in securing for another season a lease of this elegant and commodious house. As a matter of course, he has spent no end of money on the furnishing and re-decoration of the whole building. Two panes of glass which were broken, have been re-placed at considerable cost; a chair which had but three legs can now boast of four; and new gas burners have been placed in most of the brackets. No expense has been spared in increasing the stock of properties, and the services of a whole constellation of the stars of the theatrical world have been secured for the season about to commence. After such lavish expenditure, the Manager trusts that his theatre will be found second to none in comfort and elegance, and superior to many in the excellence of the performances.

The performance this evening will be under the distinguished patronage of the **RT. HON. W. E. GLADSTONE,** who will be accompanied by two Bashi-Bazouks, at present his guests in this country; the **SENIOR OBADIAH** and the **JUNIOR OBADIAH**; the **HON. MRS. W. O. EMMA,** and many more of the nobility and gentry of Cholsey and Star Terrace.

The proceeds of the performance will be devoted to supplying flannel pocket handkerchiefs to the **SWALLOWTHEWHISKIS,** a savage Central African tribe, lately discovered by Mr. H. M. Stanley, to be entirely destitute of these necessary appendages of civilized life.

At 7.30,

SHOULD THIS MEET THE EYE

AN ORIGINAL FARCE, IN ONE ACT, BY ALFRED MALTBY,

As performed by the present company,

BEFORE ALL THE CROWNED HEADS OF EUROPE

ever thought of performing it.

Characters

LAMBKIN LOUDER, (a regular Lady Killer)	....	Mr. A. Lockie.
LIONEL LONG, (who sticks at nothing in love-making)	....	Mr. J. G. Evans.
SEPTIMUS SKINFLINT, (Maud's Guardian and an old Blue-beard)	....	Mr. H. Kirby.
TEDDY, (A waiter from the Imerild Oil)	....	Dr. Barron.
NABBEM } Bailiffs	....	Mr. D. Green.
GRABBEM }	....	Mr. G. Winter.
MAUD (a sweet gushing thing of seventeen)	....	Miss Annie Hickman.
POLLY, (a charming chambermaid)	....	Miss Ellen Digby.

Scene—An Inn at Croydon. Time—The Present.

At 8.30,

THE BLIND BEGGARS,

AN OPERETTA, IN ONE ACT.

Characters.

ZACH MORGAN, { Artful Mendicants }	....	Mr. A. Lockie.
BUFFLES, {	....	Mr. A. B. Smeeton.

Scene—A Street.

Stage Manager and General Director—Mr. Lockie. Pianist—Mr. Wiltshire.

Doors open at 7. **Performance** to commence when every one is ready. **Life Boats and Velocipedes** ordered at 11. Children in arms not admitted if the arms are loaded. **Prices of Admission—Various.**

At Moulsford, posters were created for some of the regular entertainments. The posters are full of private jokes – the 'nobility and gentry of Star Terrace', for example, were the married attendants. Here, head attendant Alfred Lockie is joined by medical officer John Barron, charge attendants Henry Kirby and Ellen Digby, attendants David Green, George Winter and Anne Hickman, and porter John Evans. *The Berkshire Record Office.*

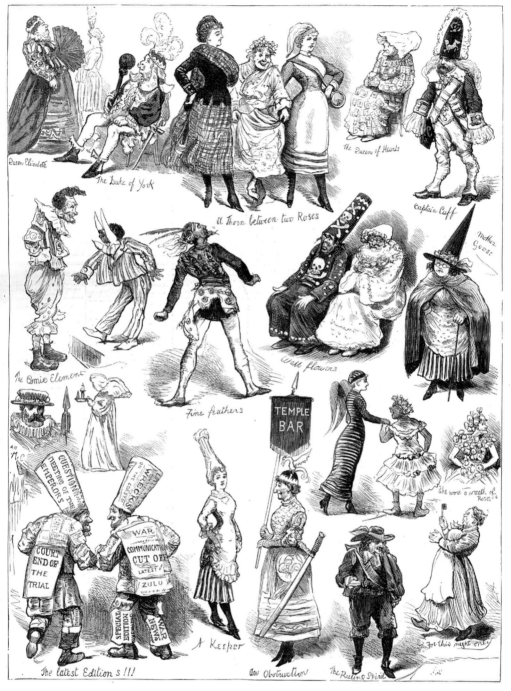

FANCY DRESS BALL AT THE BROOKWOOD SURREY LUNATIC ASYLUM.——SEE NEXT PAGE.

Patients, staff and visitors at Brookwood Asylum's New Year 'observance', 1881. The asylum band played from 7.30pm-9.00pm, wreaths and flags decorated the hall, and Chinese lanterns hung from the ceilings. Thomas Brushfield, the superintendent, is 'The Ruling Spirit' at the bottom of the image. Patients are drawn now in caricature: the sympathy of the earlier Victorian period is being lost. *Reading Libraries.*

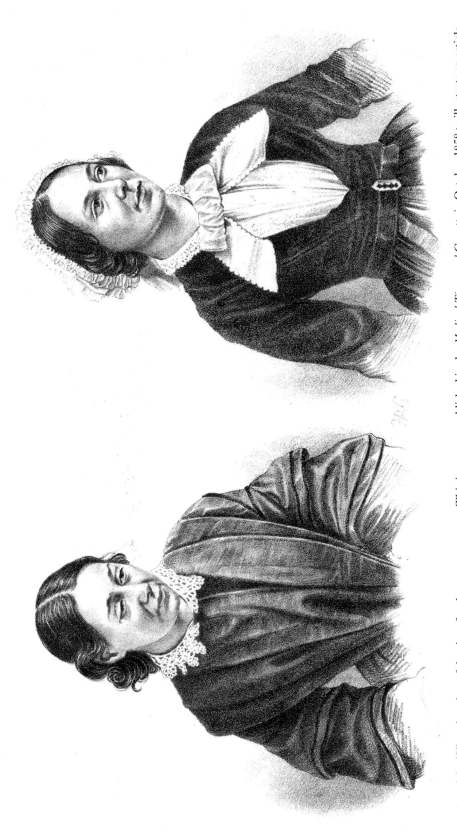

The original Victorian view of the aim of asylum care: recovery. This image was published in the *Medical Times and Gazette* in October 1858 to illustrate an article by John Conolly on physiognomy. The patient presented with melancholia linked to feelings of religious guilt. She recovered after a summer spent in an asylum. *Wellcome Library, London.*

dormitories and single rooms are closed, the bedroom doors are shut then locked. Lights are extinguished once all the patients are safely under covers. Any heat gradually dissipates and leaves a circulation of cool air, while a little glow in the dormitories remains from the lamps in the corridor and the attendant's room.

Some dormitories are watched continuously at night, especially those housing the epileptics or where any patients are known to soil their beds. Patients who are in danger of self-harm will also be under the watchful gaze of the attendant. All behaviour is monitored lest it should be offensive to others, and if necessary the perpetrators will be removed into a single room for the night, where they will be left unattended until the morning. The aim is to ensure untroubled repose, for peaceful sleep restores vitality and rationality.

Entertainments

The social side of life in the asylum is constantly promoted to the patients. Association is an important skill and easily tested in work and play, so we try and provide opportunities for large groups of patients to get together and enjoy activities across the wards. It is necessary to have a sufficient quantity of attendants on duty and so, much like the cricket games in summer, these events take place during the evenings and weekends.

Since the asylum's opening we have operated a programme of fortnightly musical *soirées*, which take place after the usual time for lights out, evoking a feeling of illicit freedom among the gathered throng. In the winter, these evenings take place in the hall, but in fine summer weather they are moved to the formal gardens outside the main block. As well as the singing and musical accompaniment, tea is available to all. It has also been found agreeable for these events to bring together both sides of the asylum. To date, no ill effects have resulted from this novel arrangement. Indeed, the benefits of this rare mixing of the sexes are of great interest to the medical men who watch over you. The most truculent man may become a lamb when faced with the gentle charms of a woman; similarly, the female patient who cannot be tamed by her sisters may submit gracefully to the orders of a male.

The music for the evening begins once the superintendent has arrived, and thereafter voices with accompaniment are heard across the estate. The music is a clarion call to dance, and the staff enquire of each patient if they would care to join the round. Some encouragement is usually required to bring the two sexes together in the hall, for they sit as self-consciously apart as participants in any parish dance. Many patients are also content merely to listen to the music.

The band itself is made up of patients and staff, and includes brass, woodwind and timpani; a piano is also available for suitable pieces. Though the musicians are amateur, the standard of playing is enthusiastic, and their steady rhythms pulse within the floorboards while their notes ascend into the evening air. Recently we have been fortunate enough to acquire an officer who has a great interest in singing, with the result that a choral union has been established. For variation, a soloist may give a rendition of some light operatic song.

We are additionally very proud of the theatrical performances that we stage. For the patients these tend to be a passive experience, as although one or two actors are drawn from the patients' ranks, for most there is rather the appreciation of being a spectator. These affairs are designed to enhance your spirits and to invite a response with their ready humour. Typically they are one-act farces with the opportunity for outlandish dress. The staff themselves can be relied upon to rehearse and perform these plays, and we offer one gala performance every two months. Where possible, these performances are also opened up to the local villagers, and a small amount of money is raised from entrance fees to go towards the purchase of dramatic, musical or sporting equipment.

The same is sometimes true of the performances by visiting artistes. The superintendent is always keen to acquire the services of at least one dramatic troupe each year, and we have occasional shows by orchestral groups, magicians and other variety acts, or lectures with the magic lantern. These artistes are amateurs for the most part or professionals who are content to waive their usual fees.

All these events are of such importance that every able patient is allowed to attend and only those too infirm to watch must sit out proceedings. They are a wonderful, shared experience: the community has a common interest in anticipating them, and then in critically dissecting the experience afterwards. There is no better sound than when the hall is awash with waves of applause or laughter.

The same privilege of mass attendance is afforded at our annual show. Each year we hold an athletics meeting one Saturday towards the end of summer. These are not the refined athletics of the university or public school; instead, it is an opportunity to enter into the spirit of taking part. Obstacle, sack and egg and spoon races are the order of the day, and the cricket pitch gives itself over to mirth and merriment in lieu of tribal competition. Involvement in the athletics is restricted to the male patients, while the women form an audience for the rustic sports that are transacted.

However, both male and female convalescents separately also make outside visits to the annual agricultural shows held locally. There the finest flowers, fruits and vegetables can be inspected, together with the most handsome beasts, while souvenirs can be purchased from the many craft stalls.

Sundays and Holy Days

In keeping with the commandment of the scriptures, every Sunday in the asylum is a special day when you may rest. You may choose to read, or write letters, play games or join with one of the walking parties.

Each Sunday we hold Divine Services within the chapel. These are much larger ceremonies than the daily prayers. A morning service commences at 11am, and an evening service begins at 6pm. The asylum chaplain is always pleased to receive anyone to the chapel, and no patient's behaviour is restrained unless it presents a danger. The services are not quite like those you may remember from your local church: the congregation is often reluctant to kneel, and it is not uncommon for patients to call out, or extend their arms rhythmically in a display of excitement. Provided that there is no harm in such displays they will be embraced as part of the character of the gathering.

There are usually around 150 worshippers at the Sunday morning service, and up to 170 at the evening one. Services err on the side of brevity, so that the attention of those present is not allowed to wander too freely. Descriptions of terror and unpleasantness are omitted from the readings and the sermons.

The chaplain is at all times requested to lift the gloom experienced by some patients, rather than to exacerbate it. Chapel is another of those rare times when male and female patients are permitted to share the same space. In some asylums there is a gallery, where the female patients sit behind and above the men, thus out of sight and of temptation. Here we have no such option, so the women merely use the rear chapel seating.

We have a small choir of patients to lead the singing at these services. Additionally, a harmonium in the chapel provides for a solid musical accompaniment to our song. Our last chaplain had complained bitterly about the 'great want which we all experience of a small organ', and it is a pleasure to have rectified the matter. Once a month, the chaplain also administers Holy Communion, though only around a dozen patients currently take part in this and specific permission has to be sought from the superintendent for a patient to take the sacrament.

There are similar, additional Divine Services on special days: at Christmas; each day throughout Holy Week; and on certain feast days, including Harvest, when a special supper is also provided. All are welcome to attend. Good Friday and Christmas day are also days when patient work is suspended. The festival of Yuletide is undoubtedly treasured by all our patients. A few days before Christmas itself, the dining and recreation halls are made up extensively with evergreen wreaths and fabric ribbons constructed by staff with the assistance of patients, while lanterns are hung from the ceilings. These bright and airy spaces are then the scene for the festivities which traditionally take place on a day between Christmas and Twelfth Night.

At these festivities every patient dines in the hall on a cooked meal of roast meats, followed by a plum or other fruit pudding; then afterwards, the merry gathering retires to the next door room for a ball based upon the programme of one of our regular musical evenings. Initially, airs are sung to a piano accompaniment, before the band is formed and the dance begins. Warm, spiced drinks and cakes are served until 10pm, when the national anthem is sung and the party disperses; but the celebrations of all are carried back into the wards.

Chapter 7

Treatment

All patients enter this asylum with the expectation of recovery. They have been sent here because we can provide treatment at the forefront of modern medical care, which is universally acknowledged as the best method of achieving respite and for cure. Much of it has already been described, as it is inherent in the organisation and workings of the asylum.

The Moral Regime

The moral regime is the bedrock of asylum life. It is based on the kindness that any man might offer to his neighbour. This kindness seeks to remove any friction that might irritate the brain, and then to influence your mind's reparation in positive ways. The object of this treatment is to subject you only to uplifting, healthy forces; it is both palliative and curative.

The first part of the moral regime – the removal of the patient from the immediate cause of illness – is the reason why your admission was recommended. This is the asylum in its proper role as a refuge from the evils of society. Your acute symptoms should subside in your new, soothing surroundings.

One might ask whether it is a kindness to detain a man so that he receives care and medical treatment? Quite apart from the statutory imperative that we are given, the detention of patients in the asylum is recognised as being the most efficient way to induce the patient to assist in their recovery. No matter what treatment is given to a lunatic outside of the asylum, there is no guarantee that he will follow his prescription, nor that his will be an environment conducive to improvement. Many men of higher birth are treated in their own homes, but that does not relieve their families and friends from the burdens of their illness. Any good physician would admit that some restriction of liberty is inevitable if a successful outcome is to be attained.

If you were very unwell at admission then you may not remember the process by which you came here or your first days under our care. This is quite common, and during such a phase we shall not attempt to practice the more active elements of the moral regime. However, once you are able to appreciate your surroundings we will begin to stimulate your mind towards the reception of healing thoughts.

Whilst the asylum is a refuge, it also promotes all that is healthy by methods tailored to suit your particular illness. With manifestations of mania, for example, the repression of strong emotion may be considered a good thing, and by discouraging manic action or expression we may discourage manic thoughts. If you are excited by the opposite sex, money or religion, then we may suggest that such topics are never mentioned in your presence. However, if you are melancholic, then it is unwise to quell emotion. Rather, we will interrupt your morbid thoughts with varied topics of conversation, thus diverting the mind from its own unhappiness.

The delusional patient requires a slightly more nuanced approach. Generally speaking, a polite but firm contradiction will be given in response to any statement of fantasy. However, staff will not attempt to argue with a delusion, for to do so is to validate its existence, and in such circumstances a delusion can only grow stronger. Instead, the right approach is to gently challenge it, wearing away at it like the tide against a stone until it is smoothed down to the smallest pebble. At this point the patient should still perceive their delusion but no longer fear it.

As you will have already gathered, physical activity and the routine of every day constitutes a great part of your treatment. Daily industrial occupation; regular meals of filling but unexceptional food; and plenty of fresh air – these are the cornerstones of your recovery. All of these elements improve the quality of the blood supplied to the brain and the strength of its flow.

It might be observed that the patient in our public asylums is afforded a greater chance of cure than the gentlemen in their private madhouses. For the food consumed by the pauper lunatic does not match the extravagant portions consumed in the private house, and the working patient obtains an industry denied to his better-off cousin. The gentleman is allowed to assume the obesity of madness while he sits before a well-stocked fire or ambles at his own pace.

In effect, the moral regime works by simply providing a distraction for a diseased mind, preventing it from fixating on its disordered thoughts. For activity keeps one's focus hard upon it and there is no time for melancholy in the dance, or for mania as the seeds are sown. These processes are rhythmic and methodical; at once soothing and calming. Their persistent application is a patient's therapy, and it will guide you ever-closer to recovery.

Of Medicines and Other Methods

It would be wrong, however, to assume that no medicine may be dispensed other than through this inspiring regime. At any one time, we estimate that around a quarter of our cases are considered curable, and so it is imperative that we use all options available. There is, indeed, much debate as to whether the moral regime has become too heavily relied upon by asylums, and if other beneficial options are wrongly avoided.

The moral regime has at its heart economy as well as practicality. Its prevalence is due to its success in both quietening the patients and in requiring only a prudent sum from the public rate. Our expenditure on drugs is relatively modest, comprising about the same amount that we spend on crops, and we strive to keep it so. Physicians can be at the mercy of sellers keen to peddle doses of some heroic new concoction, so our doctors have long understood the need to be cautious of the latest whim, no matter what the Olympian boast of the man who promulgates it. Nevertheless, occasionally other treatments will be offered if they are felt to be of worth.

Sedatives, such as morphine, are made available to calm manic patients if no other diversion is successful. Small doses of morphine dissolved into beer, wine or vinegar may be given during the day to encourage stillness, and particularly at night time as a sleeping draught. Over time, patients can even begin to recognise when they are losing control and request a dose. If morphine ceases to be effective, then chloral hydrate or Indian hemp may be substituted for it. Morphine can also be greatly beneficial to those suffering from melancholia, as it regulates their mood and brings relief from the exhaustion of their worries.

In contrast to those whose mental energy is in need of calming, stimulants may be prescribed from time to time for those in need of a tonic. Patients who are exhausted, sunken or sullen may find a short burst of new energy from spirits, while those who are weak from illness find a little brandy boosts their recovery. The only other drugs routinely prescribed are those for patients whose mental state worsens when their stomachs or bowels are disordered. Lunatics are well-known to be prone to constipation, and in these cases, purgatives such as castor oil, black draught of senna or croton oil are given to improve flow and regularity.

Dispensing is only ever done in a limited quantity. Purgatives may be decanted into bottles large enough for an attendant to administer over several days, but no more than one dose of a sleeping draught, such as laudanum, is ever issued. Accidents have occurred when attendants have been tempted to overdose the more afflicted patients.

Other treatments revolve around the use of water. If narcotics fail to induce sleep, for example, then a patient suffering from mania might be given a prolonged warm bath, while cold flannels or compresses are laid against their head. The resulting contrast between the heated body and the artificially cooled mind greatly calms the agitated man or woman. In a similar vein, patients are very rarely wrapped in warm, wet towels to stem manic activity. This is known as a 'wet pack', and is strictly limited in duration; too long an application and the towels cool, with the risk of inducing hypothermia. Cold water is generally no longer used in treatment, as it was never found to demonstrably cool hot blood; if a patient finds benefit from the application of cold water, then it is poured onto the head or upper body in small quantities, before the patient is quickly towelled dry.

In nearly all cases, these non-invasive treatments form the limits of our interventions in your malady. However, a brief word may be had on more fanciful notions, which are not entertained in this asylum but are often afoot in private medicine. It is a curiosity of the age that the private patient, perhaps due to the greater funds at his disposal, is subjected more to drastic treatments which are doubtfully substantiated by evidence.

So it is that some private houses still subject their patients to procedures long since rejected by science. Bleeding – either by cupping the body, or by the application of leeches to the temples or shaven scalp – is used in the belief that a little blood loss will relieve the worst symptoms of mania or melancholia, presumably by taking away blood considered to be overheated or chilled. An umbrella-maker admitted this year with mania showed signs of having been cut and cupped about his heart. However, there is no empirical basis for the efficiency of bleeding and we have never practised it here.

Many private doctors also remain convinced that depression can find its root in the digestive function, and as a result their patients find themselves subject not just to laxatives, but to potions that encourage vomiting or urination. The trick, it seems, is to administer just enough of the poison – typically antimony or mercury – that the patient is laid low by its effects, but not so much that he descends deeper into melancholy. Such trial and error is not something for which we have the time or inclination to attempt.

Those private patients who suffer from anxiety, and feel their heads are full of worry, can find that their illness is treated by having the skin burnt at the neck so that it blisters. The theory is that this will emit the source of their congestion. That seems a cruel enough conjecture, but even these indignities are nothing when compared to those suffered by patients who exhibit more libidinous behaviour. For although all medical men acknowledge the danger to sanity caused by masturbation, some physicians have gone so far as to blister the offending organs on both male and female patients, while the more extreme practitioners have fashioned metal prisons for the male appendage or removed the female bud. You will be pleased to note that whatever debased form your own pleasures may take, such surgery will not be practised here. A little bromide of potassium may be prescribed to slacken your desire, and your arms may be placed above the blankets pulled quite tight at night, but nothing further.

More helpful experiments – including in some public asylums – have been undertaken recently with the use of electricity. In these experiments patients are attached to a battery and a low current is passed through them. There is a growing belief that the regular application of such currents can help decidedly with cases of melancholia, though there is as yet no acceptance that the ratepayers should fund the necessary equipment.

Restraint and Other Extreme Measures

It is perhaps well now to touch upon the nature of restraint, as this measure is doubtless something that you fear. Happily, we can brush away this concern as belonging to a previous, more unenlightened age than our own. Restraint is our last resort to exercise control over patients likely to cause harm to themselves or others, and in its stead gentle coercion is always to be preferred. Many patients respond quickly to the reminder that their discharge depends on them becoming demonstrably healthy, and a simple admonishment, delivered fairly but firmly, often results in an immediate improvement in their attitude.

If persistent problems are encountered, then our normal response is to restrict privileges. While labour and fresh air are important elements of your treatment, the way in which you obtain them is not. Playing cricket or walking outside the grounds are concessions that can be removed if necessary. Should such small adjustments not yield the required results, then patients can find themselves moved down the classes of ward until they reside with the dirty and destructive. For a patient who is able to control his or her emotions, such a shock can be considerably effective.

If, due to some emergency situation, restraint has to be used, then the most common mechanism is for two attendants to take the arms of a patient, escort them towards a bench, and then sit on either side of them. Each attendant then places one hand on the patient's wrist, anchoring it to his thigh or to the arm of the seat, while one leg is wrapped around a leg of the patient. The rowdy resident thus immobilised, a situation of calm descends without fuss. A similar procedure can be adopted if the patient must be restrained upon the floor.

Mechanical restraint – that is, restraint with the use of some sort of physical aid – is viewed as barbarous, and for many decades has been practically obsolete. Only in the rarest cases, for instance where self-harm is imminent or wounds are required to heal, is such restraint countenanced. During the last decade we have had only four occasions to use it, and any incidence is of such significance that the Commissioners in Lunacy require the details to be recorded in a special book. Restraint is never contemplated lightly.

If mechanical restraint is employed then various options are available. At its simplest, restraint can be achieved by placing the patient in bed and pulling sheets and blankets or wet towels tight around them, tucking them into the frame so that they cannot be loosened easily. It is very rare indeed that we bring out the asylum strait-waistcoat, a contraption that alone cannot still a troubled patient and is also an unsubtle piece of apparatus with disturbing connotations.

There have been so few recent incidents of strapped restraint that perhaps some examples of its use might suffice to reassure you. Two spring to mind: a demented, paralytic patient whose frustrations grew into a frenzy, leading to them nearly severing an artery; and a male patient who attempted to gouge out one of his testicles. In both cases, there seemed little option but to put a temporary stop to free movement of the patients' arms.

If we fail to quell your violent behaviour through all other means and the strait-waistcoat is deployed on you, then you may also be placed in seclusion. This term is used to describe a period of isolation where you will be locked inside a single room. Unless you are at risk of self-harm, this will be one of our normal single rooms, though if you are judged in danger it may be necessary to place you in a padded room. Such an experience is apt to jolt an upset patient back towards the more normal expression of their senses.

Seclusion is less intrusive than restraint as a means of control, and it is the preferred method for coping with severe outbursts. Manic patients who shout and swear upon the wards, or who defame the Queen may find themselves dealt with in this way. Once again, seclusion is not a matter to be taken without reflection, and it needs to be sanctioned by a medical officer. Each hour spent in isolation must also be recorded and reported to the Commissioners in Lunacy, who are keen to see that it is employed only for medical reasons and never as a punitive action.

The final item associated with restraint is the rather unpleasant subject of forcible feeding. If you persistently refuse your food, yet are quite manifestly well, then the decision may be taken to intervene. At the simplest level it may be necessary for an attendant to hold your nose and then place the food into your mouth with a large spoon. If this non-intrusive process fails to work, then it is more likely that direct force-feeding into the stomach will be required.

We only resort to such enforced digestion if you are severely debilitated through either refusal or inability to take food, and it tends to be a treatment only for the most demented of our patient group. Should it be necessary, you will be placed in a chair, restrained by a sheet, and with your head rested against a pillow, before a tube is passed into your body. The old-fashioned method was to send the tube directly down the throat, though modern medicine has provided us with tubes small enough to fit through a nostril. The orifice chosen may depend upon the number of teeth you have, for a mouth full of teeth is more likely to bite down upon a tube, and wedges used to open such mouths are at risk of slipping.

Once the tube has been passed into the patient, it is customary to inject a liquid food through a syringe or to let gravity move the liquid from a bag resting above the head and down into the stomach. Fortifying fare such as port wine, brandy, eggs or beef tea are customary during force-feeding as they are easy to pass. Nevertheless, it is not a gentle procedure, and so only our most senior staff undertake it. Last year, fewer than one in twenty men and women required this remedy, and then for a duration of one to two weeks only.

Difficult Behaviours and Their Management

Having touched on the physical aspects of treatment, we must also consider the physical manifestations of mental illness. An asylum is home to the full range of human emotions and their bodily outpouring, and so painful incidents are bound to occur and need to be managed. There are three types of common event you will almost certainly witness during your stay: fits, violence and attempts at suicide.

Epileptics are always identified at admission because their fits can cause injury. Staff will enquire whether the patient has any forewarning of fits, or observe themselves whether a fit can be predicted. If so, they have an opportunity to move the patient to safety, placing them on the floor away from furniture before the rigours of a fit take hold.

Because of the special requirements of their condition, we try as much as possible to group the epileptics into their own wards. Within these wards we can provide furniture and fittings of softer material, and without sharp points, while beds and chairs can be modified so that they are lower, and closer to the floor should a patient fall. Epileptic patients can also be issued with special clothing such as hats padded with straw. Treatment for epileptics is broadly the same as for other patients, though those with very regular fits are more likely to find themselves sedated, or given bromide of potassium which can reduce the prevalence and violence of a seizure.

Epileptic fits are by far the most common form of outburst on the wards. One of the fallacies about asylums is that they are full of violent patients. This is profoundly untrue. Nor are certified lunatics more quickly provoked to violence than their non-lunatic brethren. However, where greater restrictions are placed on the freedom of a person is it always possible that violence towards their fellows, windows, furniture or staff may arise.

Not only are you curtailed here through your loss of liberty, but also through the limits placed on your freedom of choice. Your choice of diet is controlled and so too how you fill your day. Your favourite chair or bench is no longer solely yours; on hot days the shady spot outside may be already taken and in winter there may be many already warming themselves before the fire. However generous the floor space, this is a crowded, communal place and the enforced proximity to others can lead to frustration. Familiarity causes irritation and small gestures assume weighty gravity, while repetitive habits may annoy.

Some patients have additional restrictions forced upon them by the nature of their delusions. To worry about being poisoned is to become agitated by food; to hear insulting voices close at hand is to suspect your neighbour. Nevertheless, these incidents pale when compared to those brought about by the ordinary pressures of shared living. For this reason, the first response to violence is usually one of dispersal. The disturbed patient must be set free to wander in the grounds with an attendant for company, and, once calm, induced to engage in some sort of occupation. Application of the moral treatment works wonders in many cases of aggression.

If you are inclined toward aggression then you will probably be moved into a refractory ward with other patients who share that tendency. Great care is taken in these wards to remove items that may be used as weapons, though once a patient has employed a particular means of assault, this is likely to become his method of choice and opportunities can be taken to prevent similar circumstances arising: clothing can be searched for tools or cutlery; pockets may be emptied of stones.

Should you mount a physical attack you will be restrained from behind by an attendant, while if you have a weapon, an attempt is made to disarm you. It may be necessary to take away your balance with a back-heel, forcing you to fall. Once the attendants have control, you will then be restrained.

The greatest risk of harm in asylums is not, however, from other patients, but from yourself. For it is suicidal patients who exercise us more than any other, not least because of the great difficulty in accurately predicting the fatal impulse. The outward appearance of melancholia is no barometer for the true state within, and if we asked our attendants merely to watch those patients who appear sombre then we should fail to miss the carefree appearance of one who has resolved to destroy himself.

Around half our patient group will have been considered suicidal at one time or another. Those who have attempted self-murder over the past month, or before their admission, are placed in a ward where it is possible to observe them closely. What is harder to watch is whether a patient is collecting harmful items such as stones, cord, wood or metal, and for this reason bedding is regularly inspected.

The impulsive nature of suicide makes it almost impossible to guard against fully. Whilst any patient who has ever attempted it will be considered at risk of relapse, successful suicides often occur amongst those patients who have been here many years and recently shown no sign of *felo de se*. Sometimes a suicide attempt is brought about by an external factor and sometimes there is no known cause. One of our ladies could not bear to have her husband see her in her disordered condition and, as he arrived in the waiting room one day, she took herself off to the top floor of the female side, where she successfully hanged herself from a metal coat hook in the corridor. Other cases comprise another lady who swallowed a quantity of hair pins, and a man who waited until the airing court was clear before tying a noose to one of the trees.

Mercifully, we thwart the majority of attempts at destruction. Of those that succeed, perhaps the saddest case in recent years was of a young woman whose condition had improved until she was considered to be convalescing.

Soon after her move to the trusted sewing ward, she took a knife from the scullery and made off into a water closet, where she cut her throat.

If you are considered to be actively suicidal, then you will be accompanied everywhere by a dedicated attendant, even to the water-closets, and one of the medical officers will visit you daily. A form, known as a caution ticket, is also issued to all attendants looking after you, stating that you are suicidal and they must sign it to acknowledge that they have read that statement. This is usually repeated day and night at the change of each shift.

As another precautionary measure, you will be searched in the morning and evening, and helped to dress and undress. However, you will not usually be restricted in what activities you can undertake because some trust is required to encourage self-reliance. Nevertheless, we must still carefully observe you; one patient allowed to attend chapel decided to scale the holy roof, then jump; happily his fall was broken by an attendant.

Once you have recovered enough for this exceptional care to be removed, you will spend the next few months sleeping in a dormitory that is watched at all times, and you will be forbidden from being in the workshops or to work alone in the wards or gardens. It takes considerable time to regain sufficient trust for you to work with tools again.

As much as possible, the temptation to end your life is removed by deliberate design and the vigilance of staff. Attendants are instructed never to carry knives or scissors around the building; if they wish to shave, they do so away from the wards. Points of suspension are not generally found within the building: hooks, holes, poles or bars are kept to a strict minimum, and even the window shutter handles and the fittings for the gas lamps in the dormitories and day-rooms are recessed to such a high degree that no purchase can be found. Your safety is paramount.

Children in the Asylum

One of the less well-known aspects of our institution is that a small number of children are resident here, and at any time you may find a handful on our books. The juvenile patient usually stands upon the cusp of adulthood, but one or two are under ten, while our youngest was admitted at the tender age of five.

These children have come from the same place as you: a family home. They are, almost without exception, suffering from a defect in their evolution rather than a defect in their thinking. Their disabilities were usually apparent from an early age, when their parents noticed that they remained unable to control their bladders or their bowels, lacked physical co-ordination or the ability to communicate and socialise. A significant proportion are also afflicted by epilepsy.

Every family tries at first to manage these children at home, and for some this is entirely practicable, as either elder siblings or relatives nearby may provide a little extra supervision. The children here have come to us either because there are no older siblings, nor a helpful extended family, or because it has become impossible to control them in domestic life. Please do not judge their parents too harshly.

We offer these children the same treatment we offer our adult population and they are able to take a full part in the moral regime. Every attempt is also made to educate them, if their disabilities allow, from the chaplain's lessons in reading, writing, maths and scripture to opportunities for apprenticeship. Additionally, the attendants make an effort to teach everyday intercourse, as the use of a spoon or fork, or the ability to control their temper can make an appreciable difference to a child's quality of life.

Recording Your Treatment

Whatever medical treatment you undergo will be noted, beginning with admission. A new page in one of our casebooks is begun for you. Your first notes include some description of complexion, stature and gait, together with remarks on any notable facial expressions. An observation is then made of any symptoms noted before or at admission, and this maiden summary allows later comparisons to be made.

As time goes by, your case notes will be built with further observations from the medical officers, noted down during their rounds and later formally written up. The Commissioners in Lunacy suggest that notes should be made on a case once a week for the first month; thereafter once a month will suffice for convalescing cases, with one note every quarter for cases remaining unchanged. These rules are mostly adhered to, though a chronic case that has continued without variation for many years may warrant only a solitary annual note: 'No change'.

Some behaviours or occurrences may require an additional note. One of the principal features we observe is your own conduct and response to the daily necessities of life, so that any peculiarities regarding eating, social contact, speech or work will be worthy of recognition. These are the tools required if you are to successfully re-enter the community. It is important to know if you wet or soil yourself; if you reject some foods but not others; if you fail to speak in company but will speak to yourself when alone; if you hoard things or throw them away. Equally, how you respond to staff, to other patients and to your friends and family is of interest to us. Does a male patient quarrel every time he is asked to work in company? Does a female patient with infants of her own engage with children?

There is also the matter of your interest in your personal appearance and in that of others. Any fascination regarding dress will be keenly noted. The enhancement of ourselves is a key natural urge and a loss of interest in neatness or cleanliness is a symptom of an unwell mind. Similarly, inappropriate dress will be noted, as will the desire to discard items of clothing.

To these observations we add others that reflect upon your feelings and your thoughts. Though we separate those concepts, the two are much intertwined. Your disordered feelings about things such as religion, food or even people often follow from your disordered thoughts. We are always keen to observe your powers of memory and reasoning, as well as your perceptions. Of course, every man and woman in society will occasionally filter the evidence of their senses and reach conclusions that are false. Yet the difference between the sane man and the insane is the ability of the sane man to recognise and then correct his mistake. The insane patient is doomed to hunt within a false world for a truth that must elude him.

These reflections form the narrative of your case. They allow us to see how the moral regime benefits you and how your illness is progressing. They are referred to whenever your case is discussed by the medical officers or with your friends and family. They form the evidence for our actions, and the basis of our decisions.

Chapter 8

General Health and Patient Care

Although the asylum is not a general hospital, it is still concerned with bodily health and renders appropriate medical attention to its patients, usually falling under three headings: cleanliness, comfort and safety. Each one has a role to play in the running of a good asylum. As your cleanliness and comfort have already been discussed at length previously, this chapter deals with the third aspect of care: safety, and its various elements.

Medical Practice Within the Asylum

Though this is a hospital for the sick in mind, our patients are just as likely as the sane population to suffer from physical ailments. We therefore need to create suitable conditions to prevent outbreaks of disease.

Certain illnesses are more prevalent in large institutions than in other places. The first is phthisis, also described as consumption or tuberculosis, which affects the lungs, causing breathing difficulties. Phthisis is commonly found in towns where the density of population is at its greatest. This disease is airborne, which is another reason why we encourage ample ventilation throughout the asylum. For the microbes to be airborne, they must first be projected from a carrier and so attendants will forbid patients to spit into any of the ventilation grilles within the wards or onto the ward floor. Spittoons filled with sawdust are provided in each male ward and used by the patients who chew tobacco, but they are regularly emptied, then rinsed with boiling water.

The early symptoms of phthisis include a persistent cough and loss of weight. If you are found to be suffering from the condition, then you will be issued with rags to wipe your nose or mouth. These rags are destroyed once used. If your symptoms are slight you will be allowed to remain on your usual ward, but should your symptoms worsen, then you may be placed within a single room at the end of the ward corridor or even moved to the infirmary.

Persistent cleaning of the wards is the chief method by which we prevent contagious diseases such as smallpox, scarlet fever or measles. Washing and disinfecting surfaces constantly is our best defence against an epidemic. This is also true of erysipelas, the disease most prevalent within asylums, which brings with it fever, sickness and skin eruptions. Nevertheless, no amount of cleanliness is guaranteed to provide an impermeable barrier and intermittent outbreaks are inevitable. Earlier this year we had a sudden outbreak of scarlet fever, which was traced to one of the attendants' cottages.

In such cases, the infectious patient poses a grave risk to the others. Sufferers are immediately placed in isolation within the infirmary ward and all their clothing is disposed of. Each contagious disease also brings with it some peculiarities of management. Any discharge from the eyes, mouth or nose must be wiped away with a rag which is then incinerated, and a disinfectant solution sponged around the affected area, while a similar mouthwash is available for gargling. With skin diseases such as scarlet fever or smallpox, any crusts peeling from the body will be removed before the skin beneath is bathed in carbolic wash. Whatever the contagion, all bedding is changed regularly and disinfected before it is re-used.

If you are suffering from a disease then the attendants will also begin to record your symptoms, noting points such as duration and frequency of coughing or vomiting, regularity of bowel movements, temperature and pulse rates. Any unusual discharges, and also possibly urine will be collected for inspection by one of the medical officers.

Even if your illness is not catching, you may still find yourself removed to the infirmary wing, where you can be more closely observed and treated in a quiet place detached from the hurly burly of asylum life. Our infirmary is kept fully aired, but pleasantly warm, maintaining a temperature of around 60 degrees Fahrenheit. Your bedclothes will be changed regularly, while the sick rooms are also cleaned constantly, being scrubbed or wiped down with antiseptic solutions of carbolic acid diluted in water.

From time to time, the medical officers may prescribe some medicine, or even surgery for sickly patients. Emaciated or debilitated patients are often given a nutritional fortification such as beef tea. Brandy or port wine are also used: one 87-year-old male patient currently in the infirmary has been taking spirits and a hot water bottle. Sedatives or emetics are offered for physical ailments where either rest or evacuation of the bowels is required. Like other medicines, these tend to be prepared in advance as mixtures for dispensing. The medical officer decants a bottle of the mixture for issue to an attendant, who shakes the bottle before a quantity is measured out into a glass, ready for drinking. Medicine is only rarely dispensed in pill form, and if so, the attendant will first crush the pill and mix it with some food or drink.

Wounds are bathed with a diluted solution of iodine, which cleanses and also aids the healing process. If the wound is related to sores from a prolonged stay in bed or a skin complaint, then a poultice can be made from a mixture of linseed meal, water and mustard within a linen wrap. For breathing problems – such as those caused by phthisis – patients are asked to sniff steam or medicated vapours, placing their nose and mouth over a jug to inhale, and taking each alternate breath from the fumes. For patients with throat or mouth infections, gargling may be practised, though it is often lamented at how much time attendants spend teaching patients how to gargle.

More invasive treatments include the application of catheters or enemas and suppositories. Catheters are only applied to those patients who are unable to rise to urinate; a hot sponge is applied first to relax the body before the catheter passes. Enemas – for patients who are constipated or whose health would be improved by an increased level of evacuation – are supplied through an injection. Should you require an enema, you will be asked to lie on your side and to draw your knees up before warm water – sometime mixed with a little soap or castor oil – is gently eased into you. Typically around one or two pints will be used in each operation. Suppositories are introduced by hand to patients similarly positioned.

Surgical intervention is avoided unless considered absolutely necessary. If your complaint escalates, we will engage a surgeon on your behalf from amongst the local medical men and his fees will be borne by the ratepayers. The most common surgical procedures are amputations of infected limbs, or the removal of tumours found in the torso, yet a number of tracheotomies have also been performed here on patients who have attempted to cut their own throats.

Your consent, if you are capable of giving it, will be sought before you undergo any surgical procedure. Most modern surgeons use ether or chloroform gas as an anaesthetic, to ensure that you will be wholly unconscious for the operation. Of course, surgery can never be completely without risk and a successful prognosis is not guaranteed. We lost one middle-aged patient after his leg was amputated above the knee; and patients with large tumours are often so unwell that a sustained recovery is unlikely.

Emergencies

During your stay, you may witness various sudden deteriorations or accidents. Please do not be alarmed if you are party to such an event; the attendants will immediately fetch one of the medical officers and prompt remedial action will be taken. The most common emergency is a loss of consciousness. Generally, a patient who has fainted will first have their throat checked for obstructions, before their clothing is loosened round the neck and waist. Most incidents are fleeting and patients soon recover.

The greater proportion of accidents in asylums relate to falls, due to the high numbers of elderly, demented patients and also the number of patients who suffer from involuntary movements. Last year alone, a male epileptic suffered a broken leg when in a fit, while one of the female helpers in the kitchen lost her footing on a stool and broke her ankle. Falls can be upsetting to witness: cuts or haemorrhages may cause severe blood loss, while fractures may cause limbs to adopt unnatural angles. Any accident is attended to quickly, and a loss of blood dealt with either by raising the affected part of the body to let gravity take control, or else by the application of a tourniquet. With a fracture to the leg or leg joint, the patient will be comforted *in situ* until the medical officer arrives. If you have a fracture to the arms, wrists or hands, it may well be possible to place the limb in a towelled sling so that you can move around the ward until proper medical attention is obtained.

Sometimes the most tragic events can unfold in an institution of several hundred people. Water, though a vital part of our ongoing existence, can also be an agent of demise for a mind bent on its own destruction. Since we opened a small handful of patients have fallen victim to the proximity of the river. Our first loss was a 50-year-old tailor who had been suffering from a severe bout of depression. Invited to join a walking party, he used his new freedom to make for the water and plunge in. He floated on the surface for around 200 yards before disappearing from view, and when he did not emerge attendants were obliged to dredge the river in order to retrieve his body. Nor is the river the sole risk on our estate: a few years ago, a male patient fell into one of the shallow gutters which channel rainwater away from the buildings and drowned in only a few inches of water.

In such cases artificial respiration may be practised. If you have swallowed water, then you will first be placed on your front to allow the fluid to escape, then placed on your back with a pillow underneath your head, and your arms brought up until they meet above you. The arms are then brought down again and pressed against your chest. This piston motion is repeated up to fifteen times a minute for as long as is necessary.

A similar routine is practised in cases of suspected strangulation, though with the addition of cold water as a stimulant. But the sad truth is, as we have stated previously, that it is sometimes very hard to protect someone from themselves. The current male patient who has taken to hiding in the evergreens is one example. Every day he remains behind in the airing court, hoping that he will be forgotten by the staff so that he may try to hang himself from the nearest tree. An attendant is now detailed especially to check for him. And our suicidal female patient with the destructive lust for hair pins has become wont to rip them from the heads of female staff who visit her.

As we discuss the possibility of life being extinguished, it may be appropriate also to say a word about the commencement of it. Although the asylum is a medical establishment, it is not seen as a desirable place in which to usher in a newborn. Nevertheless, we are from time to time obliged to admit female patients who are pregnant. We do so only if there is no other option for their safe care. If an expectant patient is admitted, one of the female attendants will keep a close watch to ensure that no harm comes to the woman or her baby. The attendant is detailed to look out for signs of labour too, as the patient may be unaware of its onset or unable to communicate its approach.

These cases can cause great sorrow. As an example of the extremity required for admission, several years ago one patient was brought in from a local workhouse in the early stages of labour. She had begun gesticulating wildly and pulling at her hair, so much that the workhouse staff had shorn it to prevent her from injuring herself. This poor woman was held down in the female padded room until she gave birth to a stillborn child. The result of the restraint was that the mother's wrists were greatly swollen and we were unable to detect her pulse – or the absence of it. We failed to notice her own crisis, and she died later that day from complications of the birth.

Fire

A final safety warning must be raised against this great destroyer. Precautions against fire are not, of course, limited to asylums, and much effort is made within all institutions to curb the effects of unwanted conflagrations. Yet the hearth in every home is a constant source of danger, and the practices we adopt here are ones that could be projected sensibly into any domestic arrangement. Clothing is the usual culprit, and this is a particular concern for the female patients. Long dresses or hanging shawls are always at risk of ignition from a spark when a stove is opened. Such incidents usually occur in one or other of the day-rooms, and many a rug has become a blanket in which to wrap a burning patient.

As a large institution, we also recognise that we owe our patients a duty to take more formal precautions against fire. Some asylums have begun to invest in alarm systems – whereby a glass protector is broken in order to access an alarm bell – and additional staircases. Though these costs are outside our current range, they emphasise a concern for fire safety that shows no sign of decreasing. Instead, we hang a list of instructions in every attendant's room, stressing the importance of making sure that stoves are refuelled safely, closed at all other times, and put out at the end of every day. Each attendant has also been issued with a Metropolitan Police whistle to be blown in the event of fire to summon help.

We have recently constituted an asylum fire brigade from the ranks of the unmarried male attendants, who sleep within the main building. We have the latest Merryweather fire hoses, ten of which are connected to the plumbing and stowed in cupboards throughout the asylum block. Two additional portable fire pumps have been purchased from Merryweather's. This equipment was invaluable when soot from a chimney fell recently and caught fire in one of the female day-rooms; the swift application of water resulted merely in damage to a small patch of flooring.

Chapter 9

Patient Rights

Thus far our attempt to create an accurate picture of asylum life has outlined the tasks in which you must acquiesce. This suggests strongly a life of custody. You may well think of your admission as an evil that deprives you of your liberty; that gives you no say in your treatment or in your eventual disposal; and that renders you mute with others unable to hear your desires or wishes. Yet, while it is inevitable that the detained lunatic must to some extent submit, a framework does exist in which you can articulate your concerns.

You may recall that there is a statutory structure to your detention, which is overseen by the Commissioners in Lunacy, a body of august gentlemen who include members of the House of Lords, as well as experienced doctors and lawyers. We are obliged to pay heed to the rules and guidance issued by the Commissioners. The Lunacy Act ensures that they inspect every asylum annually. For two full days, a party of these gentlemen follow our rounds, inspect the wards, eat at our table and talk to patients. They then report their findings, giving a valuable evaluation of how we operate. Their reports are published so that our patient care may be scrutinised by the public.

This system of inspection does not automatically guarantee a patient voice, but it does allow for our decisions to be questioned. The Commissioners have wide experience of public and private asylums; they are able to spot poor practice and to exhort better. While their reports may offer only simple oversights – and it would be rare indeed for them to intervene in the treatment of an individual pauper lunatic – the medical officers appreciate that following the Commissioners' advice is likely to win favour.

The Commissioners judge our performance against the standards Parliament has intended or approved. A simple legal statement defines your position: you are described as a 'proper person to be confined'. There are two aspects of this definition, and both provide some ability for a patient to challenge the asylum. That you are such a 'proper person' is first evidenced by the certificates and order that brought you here. The existence of these papers, accurately completed by a qualified person, provides sufficient authority for your confinement. The medical officers at the asylum are not empowered to query this judgement and your only grounds for appeal is that the papers are incomplete or were prepared by an unqualified person.

Subsequent to your admission, this paperwork is copied and sent to the Commissioners. Unless they have reason to query your detention, the judgement as to whether you remain a 'proper person' passes to the medical superintendent here. Despite some current debate suggesting that admission should be subject to an annual continuation order, there is at present no need for the superintendent to reaffirm your suitability for care, and he is able to continue with your confinement for as long as he sees fit. At this point the nature of your confinement becomes relevant. The Commissioners' guidance suggests that you should be 'detained under care and treatment' and not for any other reason. Public protection from a lunatic is not a suitable reason for your safekeeping; rather, we are tasked with helping you to regain your health. If we fail to meet this definition then you have a right to challenge us.

Whether you choose to do so is likely to depend on your confidence. You would have to tackle the professional and class hierarchy which has already judged your interests best served by your admission here. For someone of lowly station this can be intimidating, as you must confront your fate before a rank of educated men. This rank constitutes both the medical officers of the asylum and also an extra, local level of scrutiny in the form of our committee of visitors.

The Lunatic Asylums Act of 1845 provides each public asylum with a committee of visitors: men of a certain social standing, drawn from the ranks of the local magistrates, landowners, clergy and businessmen. There is no fixed number, but our current committee numbers twelve. The chairman is also the vice-chairman of the county court of quarter sessions and he owns a large agricultural estate thirty miles south-west of the asylum.

The visitors receive an annual report from the superintendent; every two months a few of their number also make a tour of this place. Such visits are unannounced, but the visitors must see every patient, unless circumstances such as illness make it impossible to do so. They will look about your day-room, inspect your dormitory and taste your food. However, they may not necessarily speak to you unless you make effort to address them. At the end of each visit a record is made in the visitors' book, and if you made petition for your case it will be noted. The visitors will also glance at the case books and other medical records before they leave; regrettably, this is a privilege that we cannot offer you.

The committee meets more formally once a month in the board room above the asylum entrance. At these meetings it receives a shorter written report from the superintendent, which lists the patients admitted, discharged, transferred or deceased, as well as information about changes in the staff and notable incidents, accidents or enforcements of discipline. The committee members ask questions, check the accounts, and see that the rules of the Commissioners are adhered to. They act on behalf of the patients as well as for the local ratepayers.

It is to these meetings that complaints can be brought: either by patients or by friends and family on their behalf. You must inform the medical superintendent in advance if you wish to be seen by the committee. He will speak to you first, in an attempt to better understand what concerns you, but if he feels unable to resolve the problem then he will notify the committee that you wish to see them. This might be appropriate if you allege an assault by one of the attendants, or wish to criticise your treatment by the medical officers.

You will be heard by the committee at the end of their deliberations. You will be brought through the great corridor to the front of the building and taken up the staircase to the first floor. A heavy wooden door will open and behind it you will see the visitors, seated round a long table and resplendent in their fine tailored suits. South-westerly light streams brightly through the windows and onto the panelled walls, while these interested men let you stand before them and make your case.

In a recent charge of assault, a male patient stated that an attendant struck him on his chest in full view of his ward, which was assembled in the airing court. Though no bruise could be found on the patient, and the majority of the thirty-seven witnesses had seen nothing, two other patients agreed that they had seen the attendant land a blow. The patient, the attendant and three witnesses were brought before the visitors for inquisition; the attendant was cleared of any wrongdoing.

In a recent claim of ill-treatment, a young female patient – who had led a dissolute life prior to her admission – protested bitterly and unsuccessfully to the visitors for many months that she was not given medicine, before she began to accuse the medical officers of performing the most vile and immoral acts upon her. When she wrote to the visitors detailing the same accusations, they decided to interview her. They found her fantasies to be groundless.

Regardless of the nature of your own complaint, please be prepared to answer the visitors' questions; they will want to build a picture of your concerns and to examine any evidence presented. The superintendent will be in attendance to represent the asylum, and perhaps other staff or patients might be sent for. If you are female, the housekeeper will be asked to provide an opinion on your case. After all the evidence is heard the visitors will come to a conclusion. Should this go against your desires, be assured that no ill-feeling will be borne by the medical staff. A note will be made in your records; asylum life then moves on.

The Legal Status of Certain Classes of Patient

Most patients here are poor law lunatics. However, there are a handful of patients whose stay is governed by additional rules or regulations.

Private Patients

We are allowed to admit a small number of patients on a fee-paying basis. Our fees are sixteen shillings a week, slightly in excess of the amount allocated to each poor law patient. This makes private status an attractive option for families who may wish to seek respite care for a relative, or who wish to avoid the stigma associated with pauperism but cannot afford the higher fees charged by the private hospitals. Such people are mostly in the more affluent working class, and it might be said that the ravages of insanity sit more harshly on those who have some standing to protect, but limited financial choices. At the present time our private patients include a baker, a horse dealer and a brewer's apprentice; a carrier's wife, a farmer's sister and a draper's daughter.

There are limits on the number of private patients we can take. Restricted space means that there are never more than twenty at a time – a small fraction of our patient group. At times when we are full to capacity with pauper patients, those private payers must be removed to other places or returned home.

Private patients must still be admitted with the requisite paperwork, which guards against them being brought here for familial advantage instead of medical need. During the day they take part in the normal run of activities, though with the presumption that they have a choice between work or leisure. At night, they occupy single rooms. In the matter of their discharge, the medical officers may offer advice but cannot insist that a paying patient remains within our care, and a simple request from family is usually enough to grant relief.

If you are admitted as a private patient and your family subsequently find themselves bereft of funds, then you will not necessarily be removed from us. Providing that you are still afflicted by your illness, arrangements can be made to readmit you as a pauper.

Chancery Lunatics

Chancery cases are concerned almost entirely with patients possessed of significant property, and even within private madhouses they account for but a tiny fraction of those detained. We have had two Chancery patients since we opened: a pauper patient who subsequently inherited £2000 and was removed to Bethlem; and a local servant girl whose employer, an elderly blind spinster, bequeathed her an estate. If you are a Chancery patient, then you have significant protection in law. You were found insane by a committee appointed by the Lord Chancellor for the sole purpose of considering your health. This committee then oversees your affairs in society as well as your medical care, and it is to them, and the Lord Chancellor's visitors, that you must make appeal regarding your confinement.

Criminal Lunatics

Each year, some of our patients come to us via the judicial system, which makes allowance for patients suffering from mental illness to be sent to asylums rather than prisons. Such patients are termed 'criminal lunatics' by the relevant statutes.

You may occasionally have read in the newspapers or popular journals about patients ordered to be detained indefinitely 'at Her Majesty's pleasure'. The appropriate place of detention is usually Broadmoor, the national Criminal Lunatic Asylum for England and Wales. However, if these 'pleasure' patients are considered harmless then they may be received in asylums such as ours. On the books currently are several of them: a gardener who stole some wine bottles and some hearth rugs; a shoemaker who committed an assault; and a lady dressmaker who attempted suicide. They join two men transferred after spending many years in Broadmoor, both now elderly and quiet, neither of whom had committed a capital offence.

The more usual criminal lunatics that we receive have been given gaol sentences measured in months or weeks. They are petty thieves or vagabonds and are often vastly experienced in the penal system. We have a housebreaker at present; also a soldier who struck his superior officer and a widowed laundress who stole a pair of shoes. Whatever their crime and whatever their sentence, all these patients are admitted under warrant from the Secretary of State for the Home Office.

If you are a criminal lunatic, then the Prison Commissioners will pay for your stay during your gaol sentence. If you become well again then you may be transferred back to prison; however, it is common for many patients to reside with us long after their custodial warrants have expired. In these circumstances the Home Office asks the magistrates to transfer you to the pauper ranks, and you may stay here or be moved to an asylum closer to your place of origin.

Chapter 10

Discharge

Every new patient will be anxious about the possibility of gaining their discharge, and for some, this possibility becomes reality. The numbers vary, but each year around one in ten of our long-term patients are discharged, having recovered, and an even larger proportion of those recently admitted. As you enter this building, you have a one in three chance of leaving it again within your first year.

Should you be discharged, then the chances of you returning to us are small. Only around one in nine of our leavers are ever readmitted, and in these cases their attacks of illness tend to be recurrent but without a clear pattern. The happy conclusion is that there is hope of recovery for all our patients, regardless of their symptoms on admission. Last month four of our patients returned home. W.G., a 55-year-old carpenter, came in with mania after he had tried to set his house on fire. He rallied quickly and left us before the year was out. F.T., a 26-year-old painter, had been hearing voices and feared that he was being followed. He confessed freely to excessive self-abuse, and once his habit was broken his health was soon restored.

E.F., a baker's widow, also 55, had struggled to keep up her husband's business. When she feared that people wished to take it from her, she attempted to cut her throat with a blunt razor; having failed, she was discovered by her son standing underneath a roof beam with a rope in her hand. We stitched her neck wound and gave her sedatives; she regained her former self and was back home within four months. And finally, J.Bo., a young servant girl, who had developed puerperal mania after the birth of her illegitimate child, fretted that her food was poisoned. She was admitted after she jumped out of her bedroom window in an attempt to disarm an imaginary assassin. She too recovered after spending a few weeks in our beneficial surroundings.

Of course, the decision to discharge any patient is not taken hastily or without regard for their future. It begins imperceptibly as the patient is gradually more trusted by the medical and nursing staff. When you first set foot on the ward, privileges are few; however, if you are able to make progress and become a cheerful, constructive presence round the place, then a greater degree of liberty will follow. Your risk of harm – to yourself or others – has diminished. A wider range of occupations and diversions are offered to you and you may move to one of the convalescent wards.

The structure of the convalescent wards offers a system of parole. The bedrooms are unlocked at night, and the day-room doors left open to the grounds outside. Attendants need no longer accompany you everywhere and you may use the ward scullery to prepare food and drink. The *quid pro quo* is that you do not give in to mischief, wander, remove your asylum dress or engage in physical relations with a member of the opposite sex. This system of parole is effectively the first part of a trial, where you are encouraged to test the benefits of social intercourse in order to prepare you for a life outside our refuge. You will be asked to keep your bedroom tidy, to manage your personal appearance, to make your own way to work or mealtimes and to converse freely and rationally with other persons on the premises.

Assuming that this period goes well, the time will come for us to consider the practicalities of your exit. For the superintendent must first judge you to be sane, and once that great step has been taken, there are various additional factors to consider. Next we must establish that you have a home to go to. Family circumstances can change during the time a patient is under our care; new lives emerge, while others come to an end and work or financial circumstances can remove people to fresh environs.

Our task is therefore to guarantee that someone will be ready to receive you. Those who sought your admission will be contacted and an enquiry made. The Home Office likes us to provide a little extra reassurance for our former criminal patients – that the home they go to will be stable and temperate – but in all cases we do not wish to risk a repeat exposure to the triggers for your illness.

If you are a male patient of working age, we will also need to find a job for you, ideally in the same sphere – if not necessarily with the same employer – that you worked in before your admission. Male patients will need to confirm that some third party is prepared to use their labour and to pay them for it, yet female patients do not necessarily need such an external position. Instead, they may be occupied with domestic work within the home. We are also able to offer a financial benefit in the short term. For the first month of your discharge we pay a sum to your employer or your family that is equivalent to the cost of your upkeep here. This can be a great help in either expanding a workplace or simply coping with an extra mouth to feed.

Once we are happy with the situation offered to you, the news about your case is brought before our visitors, who will interview you. In his monthly report the superintendent lists those patients that he is recommending for discharge. Initially, you will be listed as suitable to leave 'on trial' only, meaning that it is possible to recall you during your first month away.

We have touched earlier on the nature of an appearance before the visitors. We appreciate that such an occasion can be intimidating, but remember to stand and do not be concerned if anxiety causes you to stammer. The interview is largely a formality, for the visitors take great delight in seeing any patient ready to take their leave. It is unlikely that they will make excessive or difficult enquiries of you, and any questions posed in your direction will be simple prompts to let you speak. After you have been heard the superintendent will invite the committee to approve his judgement, and once it is affirmed, he has the necessary authority to sanction your departure.

A set of clothes and shoes will be provided for you if you have none; otherwise, you are free to regain your own dress and possessions from the stores. With the prospect of employment, you can also feel proud that you will no longer be a burden on the ratepayers. A greeting with this news will be sent to the friend or relative that you wish to attend and collect you.

You may feel a little apprehensive at the prospect of going back to the home that you left in such unhappy circumstances. It is therefore important to remember that you return relieved of your symptoms and restored to your former disposition. If the asylum is indeed a place apart from society, as some contend, then to witness the discharge of a patient is to understand that these two worlds are not destined to be forever separate.

When a patient leaves on trial, his journey is the reverse of his admission. Goodbyes must be said in the day-room, to the staff and any friends amongst the patient group. We encourage this, for your success can serve as inspiration for your former fellows. As you travel back through the wards, past the dining room and into the great central corridor, each step takes you closer to the waiting room of your arrival. Once again, your paperwork is checked and then the senior staff will come to see you. This time, it is to offer their best wishes and to remind you that you still remain, for a short time longer, under their care.

Those who have come to acquire you may take advantage of our carriage for a journey to the railway station. The gravel on the drive may be punctuated once more by the sound of hooves, as behind you the asylum recedes into the distance. If you wish to take a backward look then you will see once more the façade of a country house peering out from amongst the trees, unchanged from your first glimpse of it.

It is impossible to predict how you will feel when your liberty is restored. We hope, of course, that you are grateful for the care we have provided; we hope also that you are not afraid. It is not unknown for patients to feel unable to cope when confronted by the world they left behind – a world which naturally provides many challenges. We suggest that you merely view this as a test and decide how you fare without us. If providence renders you unable to rejoin your previous life, then we will be happy to welcome you once again.

You are not sent away alone, for the chaplain will come and visit you once a week during the trial month. He will then report back to the medical officers with an account of how your case is progressing. During that initial month you have an opportunity to repair the bonds you shared with your friends and family, and to rediscover the skills that made you useful at your home or in the workplace. It is an exciting time, and you will cast off the limitations of the asylum routine and replace it with one more suited to your own rhythms.

After the period of trial there is the opportunity for review. Assuming that all is well, the order for your discharge will be prepared for two of the visitors to sign at their next meeting. The event of formal discharge may seem something of an anti-climax; there is no fanfare, no pomp nor ceremony. The superintendent simply makes his recommendations once again, and at the end of the committee business all his paperwork is signed. Amongst it is your discharge order. The superintendent passes the bundle of papers to the clerk, who updates his records, finding your name and inscribing in the furthest column of his registers the date of your farewell.

You have left our care.

Chapter 11

Useful Information for Patients' Friends or Family

This chapter is designed to help a patient's friends or family prepare for when a patient is admitted to the asylum. Their admission marks a significant change for you too. We recognise that you do not necessarily wish to surrender responsibility for the patient's future welfare, or to exclude them from your lives. Admission is simply a practical response to a situation that has become impossible to manage, and no one will condemn you for your role in this.

Here, we will outline how you can communicate with a patient in our care; how you can help in their recovery; and how we deal with the eventual settlement of a case.

Within the Asylum

On entering the asylum, your friend or relative will be able to receive care that is appropriate to their illness. We provide sanctuary and a routine with the best opportunities for a full recovery. Our discharge rates are quite high for those recently admitted, though there is a greater chance a patient will never be restored to health.

If your friend or relative has not returned home within the first twelve months then they may be here some time; it is worth preparing for this eventuality, particularly if you rely on the patient's income. Our advice always is to retain hope of recovery but to plan for a permanent loss.

You will see on your first visit that we operate within a clear framework of rules, because there is a printed set of them hanging on the wall of the visiting room. These rules are mostly administrative in nature, but we wish to draw to your attention the paramount importance placed upon asylum staff to offer gentleness and kindness to the patients. Care and compassion are the most basic targets for any hospital and we are proud to subscribe to them. You will find that this care and compassion is also extended to you.

Although a patient is necessarily separate from non-asylum life, you may still maintain contact with them. The principal form of contact is by letter. We realise that some of our patients and their families are unable to read or write – those numbers dwindle every year – but in such cases a member of staff will help the patient, while we hope that families can find similar assistance at home.

By law, few letters have to be communicated to patients or sent on from them. Statute insists only that we allow correspondence to pass uninspected between patients and the Commissioners in Lunacy, the Home Secretary or the committee of visitors. Outside those few individuals the matter becomes one for the medical officers' discretion. Missives are regularly inspected before being allowed to progress to their intended recipient.

An opportunity for censorship exists, though we do not withhold letters from patients purely on the grounds that the contents might aggravate them. Sometimes, the medical officers may choose to describe a letter's contents to a patient instead, particularly when the news is unhappy; but even then, the written version will be forwarded later. Neither do we withhold messages written by patients purely because the contents are confused.

We will usually decline only to send on letters if we think that the text may upset you, or if you have asked us to stem the flow of items you receive. Also, we do not censor any bulletins that contain accusations against the treatment here, and all allegations of this nature, however regular, are always investigated. It is usually a simple matter to reassure you that these charges are entirely groundless.

We realise that friends and family would generally prefer some communication from a patient than none at all, as this contact offers an update on their case, whatever the evidence of mental improvement. We hope that you will choose to write too. If so, please include details of your relationship to the patient in any correspondence and a stamped addressed envelope if you wish to receive a reply.

Visits are also encouraged. These are scheduled on the first and third Thursday of each month, between 10am and 12.30pm, and then from 2.30pm to 4.30pm, though we ask that new admissions are left to settle for a month before any trips are made. Visits take place in a designated room at the front of the asylum. Friends or relatives of any patient considered to be dangerously ill are permitted to visit the infirmary every day between 8am and 8pm.

There is no formal requirement to announce your intentions in advance, though if you are not known to us, but rather someone who has taken an interest in a case – such as the local rector, or the wife of the patient's employer – then please write first stating your desire to visit.

We recognise that visiting is not always an easy commitment, and that a day spent here will always involve some monetary sacrifice, at the very least, to cover transport to and from the asylum in addition to your loss of earnings. If you are unable to call often, or at all, then do not feel that your loved one will lack a comfort that is available to other patients. You would not be alone in finding it impossible to make regular visits.

Occasionally, we find it necessary to restrict personal contact with patients, usually in cases where a significant detriment is likely to be caused to them or when the asylum rules are in danger of being broken. You must not give a patient false hope of discharge, for example, as you risk retarding their recovery. We must also strictly control the provision of gifts, as items that contravene the required uniform or that might be used as a weapon cannot be received into the asylum. Neither are we able to store large quantities of foodstuffs, particularly perishable items. If you persist in trying to bring in forbidden goods then future meetings will be struck out.

Discharges and Escapes

If you visit a patient, then one of the topics they are likely to discuss is the possibility of their discharge. This is perfectly normal, and it does not necessarily mean that a patient is being recommended for it; no proposal will be made without you being informed. The type of discharge that we wish to see is one effected through recovery. The poor law then ceases to have an interest in the case and the state ceases to have a financial obligation towards it. If a patient is discharged to your care, then you become responsible for them and certain obligations are subsequently placed upon you.

Our first exhortation is that a recovered lunatic should not be allowed to wander, as unsupervised travel is a great risk. We would always recommend that the patient stays in the house to which they are discharged for a certain period of time. You also have a duty to be mindful of persons with whom they may come into contact. No new friend should be the cause of an unhealthy influence and neither should anyone be put at risk. This is especially true in the context of marriage; if a patient is single, then it is best they remain so. The perilous nature of a marital union should not be burdened further by the prospect of disease, and condemning future generations to similar suffering should be regarded with horror. We remain strict advocates of celibacy for the insane.

In exceptional circumstances a patient may be discharged even if they are not yet entirely well, for instance if, during the course of a patient's stay, your domestic life changes in a way that allows you to provide for their care. In this case, the patient is discharged 'relieved' rather than 'recovered'.

But discharge does not necessarily involve relief or recovery; sometimes it is not possible to bring about that conclusion. If a case turns chronic there is only a slim chance that it will ever be resolved; this is part of the reason for the recent growth in asylum accommodation. However, that very growth also means that we must sometimes consider other options for disposal of patients in our care. We are obliged to constantly review the cases here and judge whether ours is still the most appropriate place for them. If that ceases to be so, we must consider transfer or removal.

Such cases occur only occasionally. At admission, we will always check that a patient is local to us, as there have been incidences of wandering persons brought here whose proper place of residence is distant. In such cases, it is entirely proper for relatives to petition this institution for transfer to another, more local asylum. More significantly, there are times when our own institution approaches its capacity and it is necessary to board patients out in other houses. Usually the quieter and easier to manage chronic patients are selected for such temporary arrangements, particularly those who have no recent history of visits from friends or relatives.

As the question of removal arises, it is advisable to address the matter of unauthorised discharges too, by which we mean an attempt made by the patient to escape. There is a very strict definition as to what constitutes an escape: a patient must make their way outside the asylum grounds and in so doing, fall out of the sight of staff. Any such event is noted, yet it is a comparatively rare occurrence – we suffer between two and three attempts every year, and patients are almost always retaken quickly. Nevertheless, it is best avoided: many patients are unable to make their way safely, and are at risk of harm from the road, the railway or the river. An escape is fraught with danger even if – as in our most recent case – the patient is later apprehended sitting peacefully in the family home.

In a situation like this your help becomes vital. Should a patient arrive at your domicile unexpectedly, please make immediate contact with your local poor law officers, who will take the necessary steps to escort the patient back to the asylum. Once they have been returned, we will review the ward on which they are accommodated; a short period of time within a more secure ward is often recommended, and privileges will also be withdrawn.

Please also be aware that if more than fourteen days elapse between escape and recapture, then the warrant authorising detention becomes invalid due to the limitation periods prescribed by the Lunacy Act. Should you wish to secure a readmission, you will have to lobby your local poor law officers and construct all the necessary paperwork once again.

The Death of a Patient

Sadly, death is a common resolution to most of our patients' time with us. On average, somewhere between one in seven and one in ten of our patients will die each year. This may appear a high figure – and is a fact not noised about to the patient group – but it is inevitable that a place of long-term care should produce such figures. As far as possible, we ensure that death occurs away from the busy wards and within the quieter infirmary area.

Staff are well practised at recognising the onset of a final illness and perform the necessary removal of a patient quickly and without fuss. All patients are given peace and privacy at the end, and additional comfort can be provided through the prescription of sedatives.

We will communicate with you whenever a patient becomes gravely ill, by telegram should the end be imminent. If you are unable to visit then we will keep you informed as to how matters progress. If the patient has outlived their friends and family then we shall endeavour to make contact with more distant relatives.

Certain practical procedures must also be followed whenever a patient dies. The first duty we perform is to conduct a post mortem examination, as any previously undetected injury or disease can be discovered and also there is an opportunity for medical research. All organs are examined and weighed, while the shape, colour, clarity and consistency of the brain are investigated. The results may be contributed to a medical journal or compared with current literature.

Your consent to a post mortem is not required, though the superintendent can consider limiting its extent. It may be considered prudent to leave the head of the deceased intact, for example, should you wish to arrange an open casket before burial. Please inform us if you wish this to be done.

We are also obliged to inform the local coroner of any death within the asylum, and to make a statement verifying whether or not the circumstances of the death were unusual. If they were – or, more properly, if the coroner considers that they were – then it is likely that an inquest will follow on our premises (rather than in a tavern, as is customary). The coroner has the power to call witnesses, and will wish to hear from those who were in immediate attendance on the deceased shortly before their death.

Once the body is released for burial, two of the attendants will lay it out. The patient's eyelids are closed and a bandage is applied to support the lower jaw, while the limbs are straightened with the arms placed neatly at the deceased's sides. Further bandages bind the ankles and the toes; whatever clothes the patient was wearing are removed; the body is washed and then dressed in a clean sheet. This is how your friend or relative will be presented should you wish to reclaim their body for burial. That option is not without expense, as you will need to pay for collection and transport as well as the costs of a private interment, and for this reason most of our patient's bodies are not reclaimed. There is no shame in this; many families find themselves obliged to invest their limited resources in the living, rather than the dead.

We can offer our deceased patients a peaceful plot in the parish churchyard some two miles from here, and within walking distance of the local railway station. Our original plan was to have a cemetery within the grounds of the asylum, but the Commissioners in Lunacy felt such an arrangement would be morbid.

The Norman church by our burial ground is very picturesque and lies a little way out from the centre of the village. The space reserved for the asylum burials is delineated from the rest of the burial ground, sited on a large and open, grassy space, containing iron grave markers. Headstones have been ruled out by the visitors on the grounds of cost. If your friend or relative is to be buried here then we expect that a memorial will not be a pressing concern for you.

The End of Your Relationship with the Asylum

So it is that every lunatic is called away, and the asylum gates are closed behind them. With death or discharge also comes the end of your relationship with our asylum. Any possessions belonging to the patient can be collected or disposed of as you wish.

We have done our best to improve the part of the patient's life that they spent here, and offered compassion and security to every sufferer. We have employed the latest treatments in all our efforts for recovery.

One final word of caution: modern medicine is yet to reach a conclusion as to whether mental illness is infected with a hereditary taint passed within the blood. The risk to other family members may be greater if a relative spends time within our care. While it is unlikely that we will ever see you again, perhaps you might like to keep an eye on those within your close family for symptoms of similar afflictions. And please do ensure that someone keeps an eye on you.

Part II

The History of the Victorian Asylums

Chapter 1

Moulsford Asylum:
The Inspiration for this Book

The Victorian asylums were real places, and they existed in exactly the way I have just described. Public asylums opened across England and Wales throughout the nineteenth century, and any ordinary Victorian man or woman would have been familiar with them. These institutions were a remarkable monument to a belief in welfare, although they were not universally acclaimed; and ever since they opened, people have argued about the effectiveness and desirability of them.

I have sought to recreate the workings of a public asylum as it operated during the last three decades of Queen Victoria's reign. My model was a rather small and insignificant county asylum but one that is very dear to my heart, because it is local to me. It still stands beside the A329 between Reading and Oxford, and is remembered now by the name of Fair Mile Hospital, though it was built as the Moulsford Asylum. Technically, it was the first (and only) Berkshire county lunatic asylum, though that latter name was seldom used.

Berkshire was a latecomer to the provision of public asylums. Although the local justices, who were responsible for county government, had considered a joint venture with Buckinghamshire and Oxfordshire after the 1808 Asylums Act, nothing came of it. When Berkshire, like all counties, was compelled by the 1845 Asylums Act to provide some sort of facility, the justices decided to contract out provision to Oxfordshire instead. This was because the neighbouring county was building its own asylum, Littlemore, at Iffley, on the southern outskirts of Oxford.

Soon after Littlemore opened on 1 August 1846, Berkshire concluded an agreement for the admission of its own patients. The county financed two wings at Iffley, one male and one female, to house the Berkshire lunatics.

Along with every other English county in the Victorian period, Berkshire then experienced an unplanned increase in its number of admissions. Before twenty years had passed, the growing pressure on the space at Littlemore forced the justices to board out patients in other places, including at the Dorset Asylum and a private house in Camberwell, neither of which were close at hand for the families of those transferred. It was also very expensive to manage contracts with so many different providers; and the unexpected complexity of these arrangements led the Berkshire justices to conclude that it might be simpler to create their own facilities.

Building Moulsford

In the spring of 1866, an advertisement was placed in the Reading newspapers, requesting offers of land for sale which would make an appropriate site for a new asylum. The justices received just two, which was not so much a case of local antipathy but a reflection of market forces. There was little money to be had from selling land to the county, and unless a landowner needed the money quickly, he would be better advised to sit tight. Nor was it guaranteed that an offer would be deemed suitable, as the county was obliged by statute to look for that 'airy and healthy situation' prescribed by Parliament.

Fortunately, one of the two sites offered was almost entirely suitable. It cost the justices the princely sum of £8,000 to acquire, and comprised around eighty acres in a rural area on the edge of the Berkshire Downs. This estate was located nearly twenty miles north-west of the county town of Reading, about a mile from the small village of Cholsey and the same distance from the nearest Great Western Railway stop. Its proximity to the latter gave the new venture its name. Indeed, the Railway Hotel at Moulsford hosted lunch for the Berkshire justices after they had viewed the fields they were about to purchase. While they dined, these county men decided to plan an asylum for 300 patients.

The project was a partnership. The county joined with the boroughs of Reading and Newbury and the costs were apportioned according to how many beds each party required. The Gothic designs for Moulsford were drawn up by Charles Henry Howell, a well-known architect of Victorian asylums and later a consultant to the Commissioners in Lunacy. Howell had just finished work on Surrey's Brookwood Asylum, near Woking. The principal contractors were Mansfield and Price of Holborn, London, and they were given a little under £50,000 to complete the work – comparable to around £20 million today.

Some other facts and figures about the initial building at Moulsford give an insight into the size of a Victorian asylum. The first delivery of materials alone consisted of 900,000 red bricks, 9,000 feet of 'Baltic timber' (beech, ash or pine), and 1000 individual sections of iron rainwater goods. The scale of the enterprise was immense. Rather than use the railway for delivery – which would have necessitated an additional short journey by road – a miniature tramway was laid between the construction site and the River Thames, which formed the eastern boundary of the site. All the materials were delivered by barge and then dragged by horse along the rails.

A team of 230 labourers were permanently engaged on the project, with another 50 or so joining for the spring and summer months before leaving for the harvest. Even with such a large workforce, it took around a year to get the main building watertight, and another year to complete its internal fitting out, which demonstrates how much work went into the fixtures, joinery and decoration and suggests that the quality of these institutions did not end at their elegant façades.

The building thus created was the one on which the description in *Part One* of this book is based. Once complete, it had capacity for 285 patients – slightly below the original estimate – with 222 of those sleeping in dormitories and 63 in single rooms. It was divided up as I have outlined, by sex and by block.

Inside, £9,000 was spent on fitting out the wards to reflect the latest in Victorian conveniences. The grounds too were carefully designed for their purpose. Robert Marnock, an experienced landscaper, was briefed to provide a calm and restful space. His blueprint placed specimen trees and shrubs within a wide lawn.

Moulsford opened on 30 September 1870, and was immediately tested. As the initial batch of patient transfers were concluded, it was discovered that the group from the Dorset Asylum came complete with head lice, which they duly transferred to everyone else. Then, within two months of opening, a more serious predicament arose: virtually all the plaster ceilings in the main block gave way, and large parts of the building were evacuated. Mansfield and Price were called upon to rectify the situation and the remedial work bankrupted them.

Six months later the re-plastered asylum was able to recommence admissions, and the rest of its early years were free from similar disasters. Moulsford was comparatively set fair for a trouble-free existence: not only was it relatively small for a late Victorian asylum, but the rules and regulations for the management of such places were by now well established. All the staff had to do was stick to the rulebook and things were likely to run efficiently.

Staffing the Asylum

For many years, historians assumed that the Victorians saw asylum work as low-grade, and likely only to attract applicants unable to secure better employment. The picture generally painted was of an economically excluded staff in control of socially excluded patients. However, the Moulsford archive tells a different story, suggesting that the asylum could compete for labour with other employers. Although it did not necessarily offer the best terms and conditions within the marketplace, it offered the security of a permanent position in a growth industry, as well as opportunities for training and promotion. Indeed, you can follow some of the more high-flying Moulsford staff as they moved around the asylum network in pursuit of betterment.

What is certainly true, however, is that the work was not to everybody's taste. It could be physically hard and emotionally challenging. There were high expectations of the attendants on the ward and every year a reasonably high proportion of the staff would decide they could no longer meet them. This problem was compounded by the presumption that single female staff should resign upon their marriage.

At the top of the staffing pyramid, Moulsford's Victorian superintendents were all wedded to public service. The first of them, Robert Bryce Gilland, had served his apprenticeship in the Glasgow Royal Asylum before he moved south to work in the Essex Asylum at Brentwood. He was 32 when he took charge of Moulsford, and he negotiated an initial salary for himself of £300 per annum, also securing an extra £600 to furnish his quarters.

Gilland was the superintendent whose breakdown fifteen years later is referred to in *Part One*. His demise was gradual but spectacular, and begs questions as to what extent the committee of visitors tried to hold superintendents to account; surely Gilland's problems might have been spotted before the asylum lost such a high proportion of its management in quick succession? Gilland was also the first in a line of Moulsford's leaders to die in post; a similar fate befell his successor, Joel Harrington Douty, though in Douty's case it was simply bad luck rather than overwork, as he caught a chill and died suddenly in 1892 at 34.

Upon his death, deputy John William Aitken Murdoch took the reins. Murdoch was another Scot, a native of Dumfries who had previously worked at the Paisley Asylum. Unlike Gilland and Douty he married, though in keeping with Victorian protocol he waited until after his appointment as head doctor. His bride, Celia Cozens, was the daughter of a local farmer.

Murdoch was the last superintendent of Victorian Moulsford. He remained in charge until 1917, when he died at the age of 60 following an operation in Reading for appendicitis. Murdoch did far more than his predecessors to improve his staff's rewards in terms of allowances and leave, and it seems reasonable to assume that Moulsford was a happier workplace under his command than under Gilland's micromanagement. Murdoch's most remarkable legacy is, perhaps, not at the asylum itself, but at its cemetery in the village churchyard. There, within the otherwise featureless plot containing the graves of his patients, is a splendid stone angel, once blowing a now-lost trumpet. The inscription beneath the angel reads 'Write me as one who (laboured for) loved his fellow men the angel said', and underneath it are the superintendent's remains and those of his wife. Murdoch evidently intended to look after his patients in death just as he had in life.

These three superintendents had a small staff that befitted the compact nature of the establishment. The forty staff in 1870 grew to around sixty by the turn of the twentieth century. There was a reasonable amount of continuity in all the senior posts, with the exception of the role of chaplain. The high turnover in that role illustrated its lack of desirability to clerical job-seekers. Most chaplains went onto better things, with two becoming the local parish rector; the philandering curate, Frederick Agassiz, was an unusual case of an incumbent who chose a less respectable career. Agassiz ended up in Massachusetts, while his misused wife was eventually obliged to divorce him.

In contrast, the posts of steward and housekeeper enjoyed the greatest element of stability, perhaps helpfully as these were arguably the two persons most crucial to the smooth running of the operation. The first steward, Edwin Stott, came straight from the rank of sergeant major in the Royal Lancers, while his successor joined from a role in the office at the Wiltshire Asylum. The first housekeeper, the widowed Hannah Horton, also began work as part of Gilland's original team and was one of the senior staff who resigned just before the latter's breakdown – the other being John Barron, Gilland's assistant medical officer.

Although I have referred only to a head male attendant, Moulsford went on to employ a head female nurse as well as the housekeeper. I did not describe this role separately in *Part One* because the role of head female attendant took time to evolve, and even by the turn of the century still did not perform the range of duties granted to the head male attendant. Moulsford also had an extremely long-serving head attendant, a gentleman called Alfred Lockie, whose employment spanned virtually the entire Victorian period and whose longevity demanded recognition in this book. Lockie was the navy pensioner who had worked previously at Cambridge Asylum, then joined the Moulsford staff in 1874 and remained in Berkshire until his retirement in 1903.

A photograph purportedly showing Lockie still exists. It depicts a squat, generously-built man, who also manages to look wiry and strong; his hair is greased back, though his curls are trying to break free at the back. This provides a flat surface on his head in contrast with the wild, bushy quality of his generous beard and whiskers. His eyes are narrow but his face has a benevolent quality, like a village policeman who has admonished a cyclist for riding on the pavement, and is now watching the same bike ride away.

That look tallies with what Lockie and his attendants were trying to achieve: a regime that was both custodial and restorative. The staff were expected to live and breathe their work, with single staff obliged to live in, and single or childless applicants preferred for most posts. The close proximity of staff resulted in strong bonds being formed, and workers were very quick to support each other.

For example, when one attendant died shortly after the birth of his first child, a collection was immediately gathered for the benefit of his widow. A year earlier, in 1875, a popular attendant, James McLaren, had suddenly been taken very ill. When it proved impossible to find friends able to care for him, he was simply admitted to the asylum as a patient, where he died from what was described as 'acute brain disease'. Gilland wrote: 'this unfortunate man…was industrious, sober and a very good attendant…a large party of fellow servants followed him to the grave'. A stone cross was erected to his memory in Cholsey Churchyard.

This support was balanced by the expectation of discipline. Any staff who did not follow the asylum rules were likely to be punished and their misdemeanours, no matter how inconsequential, recorded for posterity in the superintendent's report to the visitors. This is how the story of the porter's drunken night in town has been handed down.

That is not to say that all transgressions were equally humorous in nature. In May 1871, 26-year-old Hannah Mulcay, a laundry maid, was found one morning with a blood-soaked shawl by the side of her bed. It transpired that Hannah – who had recently 'got stout' according to Mrs Horton – had given birth to an illegitimate child during the night. She claimed it was a miscarriage, but then the body of the full-term baby girl was discovered, wedged behind the hot air pipes in the drying room. Hannah was charged with murder, though she was convicted only of the lesser charge of concealment of a birth. She was sentenced to six months' imprisonment and her final month's wages signed over for the use of Reading Gaol.

A regime of summary dismissal existed across asylums. If you were discovered asleep or drunk on duty, struck a patient or went absent without leave – like the Moulsford carpenter and asylum band leader once did to play a concert in Wallingford – then you would be asked to leave the establishment immediately, without the necessary references to recommend you to a future employer. Although there was technically a right of appeal to the visitors, few staff took it. The superintendent's word was law.

The Patients' Stories

That quality of law is apparent also in the patients' case notes, which record the medical officers' observations on every man and woman under the asylum roof. In these notes people's lives are reflected over a period that, for many, amounted to decades spent in Moulsford's care. Compassionate paternalism is probably the kindest way to describe the medical officers' approach to their charges. They were certainly wholehearted believers in the recuperative power of their regime, and also quite convinced that they knew best.

This is visible too in the occasional incidences they encountered of patient non-compliance. In 1896, for instance, the husband of a female patient, Ruth Noakes, visited and noticed a bruise on her. Incensed by what he considered to be evidence of abuse, Mr Noakes began to strip his wife in the visiting room, despite the presence of a handful of male patients. When a female attendant tried to intervene he abused her and maintained his accusation.

Dr Murdoch was sent for and heard out the complainant. Murdoch defended his staff, refused to take any action and then wrote a note summarising his investigation: 'Mindless, mischievous woman who is constantly getting into trouble with the fellow patients. She is very impulsive and amorous starting up and trying to embrace other patients. The more irritable of these quickly retaliate but the more sensible grip her by the arm and put her down on her seat. Being a toneless and flabby woman the slightest pressure leaves a bruise...Her husband has not visited since the August bank holiday (a special privilege) and he was drunk then.'

This rather dismissive approach could create problems at times. The poor woman in the padded room, who was restrained while she gave birth – and whose plight was described in *Part One* – was one such case. Harriet Harpwood was a 28-year-old labourer's wife from Abingdon, and the stillborn child she gave birth to was her fourth baby. Because Harriet's involuntary movements were both constant and violent, the medical officers had concluded that the padded room was the only safe place for her. Three mattresses were put down for her to lie on as she gave birth. Harriet's grave state passed almost unnoticed until it was too late, and the death of both mother and child seems to have shaken the staff. Her only comfort had been the presence of her husband at the end, and the fact that she seemed 'evidently grateful' for his presence.

Some of the more robust attempts at treatment were also not without their risks. Mary Belcher, a housewife of mature years, had begun to see visions of angels and also to suffer from the common delusion that her food was being poisoned. Refusing it, she was force-fed up to three times a day for many weeks. After one such bout of treatment she was persuaded to eat a dinner of beef, carrot and potatoes. A piece of beef wedged in her windpipe and she choked to death within five minutes. The trauma of eating solid food after several weeks of the liquid pump cannot have helped.

However, such incidents were rare. Force-feeding was about as unpleasant as physical intervention could get, while restraint of any kind with clothing or sheets was seen as a recourse only after the failure of other measures. Rather, staff were encouraged to interact with the patients; and the routine of industry, fresh air and regular, bland food was intended to build up patients' health. Moulsford was the very epitome of Victorian lunacy reform. Each recovered patient was proudly paraded before the committee of visitors and each annual report made great play of its proportion of discharges.

There are many uplifting stories amongst the patient group, suggesting perhaps that the therapeutic environment was of benefit to some people. Grace Borlace, a middle-aged housewife who was admitted with profound melancholia, was convinced that her husband intended to kill their children, and also paranoid that he was keeping a pig in the house to upset her. She was barely sleeping and took no interest in life or her own appearance. A few months' rest at Moulsford seemed to do the trick: she was discharged recovered shortly after.

It was a similar tale for Sarah Cannon, who is one of the patients mentioned anonymously in the chapter on diagnosis (see the notes at the end of this book for a complete list). Sarah was 28 when she was admitted with 'exhaustion caused by suckling her child for two years'. She had tried to kill her husband at home in Maidenhead and separately attempted to strangle herself with her stockings. At Moulsford, she found herself consumed by sadness during each week's divine service, but also that occupation and work provided relief of her symptoms. Once she was restored from her 'prolonged lactation' she was sent back home.

A browse through the Moulsford case notes certainly proves the Victorians' keenness to attach mental illness to critical, hormonal phases of life. Puberty, pregnancy and the climacteric menopause all feature regularly on the female side, while procreation and provision – career and money matters – are the chief equivalent male maladies. These reasons for admission are interspersed with accidents, illnesses and personal catastrophes: the sorts of things that fill doctors' waiting rooms today. Reading through Victorian case notes makes you realise how timeless mental illness is.

What has changed, however, is that now we recognise mental illness and learning disability are not the same. Victorian doctors knew that, but wider society was slow to differentiate, and this explains why a handful of children were sent to Moulsford before 1900. It is difficult now to conceive of sending a child to the asylum, yet such decisions were felt to provide the best quality of life possible for these individuals.

Most of the cases followed a similar pattern: the disabled child was born into a family with many brothers and sisters. The disabled child's behaviour was disruptive and made nurturing the other children difficult. Despite that, the parents had resolved to manage their child's condition at home. They continued to do so until they considered it impossible, usually when the child reached puberty and became physically stronger and therefore harder to discipline. By this stage, the child had slipped far away from formal education and was living what must have been a fairly basic existence at home, unable to compete successfully for love, care or intellectual stimulation. The child was then sent to the asylum in the hope that more attention could be given to them. They would also find open spaces which might be more practical than the confines of home.

Only very rarely were these children under 10 years of age. The youngest child in Victorian Moulsford was little Frederick Freeman, who was the son of a journeyman plumber from Wantage, and just five years old when he was admitted in 1878. His parents told the medical officers that they had considered him to be a bright boy until he suffered some sort of seizure at the age of two. Afterwards, his progression ceased: he became unable to control his bladder or bowels, he tore around the house breaking things and frequently attacked his four brothers and sisters. His mother resorted to tying him to a kitchen chair to subdue him.

In contrast to those limited conditions, Moulsford must have afforded Frederick some degree of liberty as well as care. His notes suggest that the staff taught him to speak a little and how to use the toilet, while he gradually became able to feed himself. It reads as though he gained a little dignity. However, the unsuitability of leaving a child in an adult's world was also apparent, as Frederick would spend most of the day sat in the day-room, drooling, and sucking at the corner of his oversized asylum jacket. At night, he cried – every night, for eight years. Over time his fits increased in violence and duration, and he died at the age of 13 in 1886.

Thirty Years of Evolution

Between 1870 and 1900 Moulsford was a very typical Victorian asylum. Because it was rather small and unglamorous, though, it never attracted the finest medical minds, nor was it ever home to great clinical or management innovations. On the other hand, there were no real scandals uncovered by the Commissioners in Lunacy and no significant criticisms of the asylum's practice. Moulsford simply got on with its job.

Locally, the new county asylum was of great economic benefit. The nearby village of Cholsey grew from a population of 1,300 to around 2,000 in those 30 years; an increase that ran counter to the rural depopulation seen by neighbouring parishes. It was quite clear that asylums contributed to growth: tradesmen and retailers set up close to the institution, which sourced almost everything locally; there was a large degree of interaction between the two communities. The villagers became used to seeing walking parties of staff and patients filing over fields and round the country lanes; they played games against the asylum teams and formed the audience at the asylum shows. The staff married in the parish church and their children went to the church school, while patients who died at Moulsford were buried in the village cemetery. It was hard to separate the people within the gates from those without.

That physical divide is worth reiterating because of the impact it had on asylum management. One task of maintaining the Victorian establishment was ensuring that patients were only discharged when you wanted them to be, which was not necessarily straightforward with an occasionally reluctant group. It took time and the experience of escape attempts to hone security on the large, sprawling site. There were regular efforts to abscond, usually by patients making over the walls of the airing courts or running off while walking in the grounds.

Only rarely were these attempts successful. Most patients could be easily outnumbered by pursuing staff, who were able to take differing routes to head off their quarry. Security was improved by detailing two attendants to lead each walking party; by moving the airing court walkways further away from the walls; and by increasing the number of locked doors. Just one route remained impossible to secure against a successful escape, and it was not without risks.

I noted earlier that the site for Moulsford seemed almost entirely suitable, and so it was. The only thing not at all suitable was its location adjacent to the River Thames. Having a river for a boundary was very much a mixed blessing, as for some patients, the perpetual flow was a deterrent to escape, while for others, it provided an excellent opportunity for the quest of liberation.

Sometimes there was a comic element to escapades within the running water. In January 1873, patient James Lemon bolted from a walking party in one of the airing courts and took off into the surrounding fields. There was a determined, if low speed chase across the meadows, before a group of attendants caught up with Lemon and surrounded him on the river bank. Lemon paused, took in the rather hopeless nature of his situation and then jumped into the ice cold winter currents. He proceeded to swim, rather competently, upstream. However, none of the attendants could swim, so they were obliged to watch as their patient made a smooth getaway. After a moment's pause the staff realised that their best bet was to make downstream, where the Moulsford ferry offered a route to the other bank. By the time the little boat reached the Oxfordshire side, the attendants found that a passing labourer had snared their prey. The ferry made the return trip with Lemon aboard.

At other times the river delivered tragedy, as recounted in *Part One* of this book. Robert Warren was the 50-year-old tailor from Reading who became the first to perish in this manner. He had always refused to go out walking round the village on the grounds that he was 'well-known in Moulsford', but after lobbying from his wife was allowed instead to join a small party walking in the river meadows, with fatal consequences. His demise was rare but not unique. William Goodyear had been in the asylum for nine years when he made a similar leap in the spring of 1879. The river was in full flood after persistent rain, turned brown by mud as it sped along the valley. Goodyear's body was found five miles downstream seven days later.

Such horrors were the exception to asylum life. Soon after its opening Moulsford settled into a gentle routine, and the activities of the moral regime punctuated each day, while the seasons were marked by outdoor sports or indoor entertainments. Every ward was always full of patients and there was also a constant pressure from the workhouses to admit more. Within seven years, the first extension was planned to virtually double the asylum's capacity to 535 beds.

The Moulsford experience suggests that the medical officers were reluctant to expand their empire. That first extension was prolonged and painful, delayed by a severe winter in 1878-1879 and then saddled with overcrowding on the male side while some wards were given over to the builders. Patient death rates increased noticeably, the presence of the builders curtailed the regular entertainment programme and the constant turnover of strange faces upset the patients. There must have been relief all round when the new recreation hall and enlarged day-rooms were finally completed at the end of 1880. The hospital had also taken the opportunity to install gas cookers in the kitchen and to build a separate infirmary building, so that contagious cases might be isolated.

Not all the vast increase in capacity was utilised immediately, so Moulsford was able to sell some spare beds to other asylums and make a little extra money. It also expanded its intake of private patients. This measure, and funds left over from the extension project, were put towards building a large and impressive greenhouse to offer a better range of summer produce and for bedding plants. A ha-ha was constructed too; though almost at once, one patient fell over it, breaking several bones.

The growth of the institution led to other changes: more pathways were created for walking; a herd of sheep was purchased to live with the cows and pigs on the farm; more attendants were hired (and for the first time, given a uniform allowance); and greater mechanisation was introduced to the laundry. A telegraph system was introduced, connecting the main buildings to the superintendent's house and all the staff cottages. At about the same time, it was also decided by the Great Western Railway to move the local station from its original position on the Reading road to a site next to Cholsey village, a shorter distance from the asylum. Such was the economic power of the institution.

The demand for beds never stopped. Harrington Douty laid the blame for the increase in the patient group at the door of modern Victorian living. He wrote in 1888 that 'we have to deal here, in the main, with insanity resulting from family taint, from general bodily diseases, and from an insufficiency rather than an excess of the luxuries of life.' Put simply, his patients were poor people with limited life chances, and unless the causes of insanity were tackled, the insane would always be with us.

Douty was still in charge when the Lunacy Act of 1890 replaced the earlier legislative framework governing asylums. In theory, this Act tightened up the law on admissions – causing Douty to complain about the additional paperwork now required of him – but it did nothing to stem the influx of patients. Perversely, other legislation even instituted the payment of a premium to the poor law officers for each person relieved via the asylum rather than the workhouse. The scene was set for further demands on Moulsford.

When James Murdoch ascended to the post of superintendent there was pressure once more on space. Murdoch described how attitudes had changed since his institution opened: 'asylums are looked upon as nursing homes for the demented and aged, and as houses of detention for idiots and imbeciles', he wrote in 1896. The idea of the asylum as refuge, dispensing specialist care was being bypassed. By now, the existing buildings at Moulsford had been rearranged to squeeze in another 100 patients and, as the borough of Windsor was due to join the partnership the following year, a further extension was planned.

By the time that second extension was complete, at the beginning of the new century, Murdoch's asylum had 800 beds, some three times the size of its original design. Linoleum covered the wooden floors, electricity was taking the place of gas, and communications were now made by telephone. It was a radically different place to that first conceived by the Berkshire justices in 1866. In time, that legacy would move the concept of the Victorian asylum even further away from its creators' intentions.

Chapter 2

A Word about Broadmoor

Berkshire has another asylum. Still in use, it is located on the southern edge of the county, next to the village of Crowthorne, having opened in 1863 as the national Criminal Lunatic Asylum. Its name, of course, is Broadmoor Hospital, and it has also informed the contents of this book. Though my physical descriptions of the wards and gardens may be of Moulsford, various elements of Broadmoor's history are also included in *Part One*.

This is entirely fitting, for Broadmoor was run on the same basis as any other public asylum. It was constructed on the same principles, employed staff who obeyed the same rules, received patients suffering the same symptoms and then subjected them to the same moral regime and treatments. It was simply a bigger, more secure version of Moulsford, also governed by the regulations dispensed by the Commissioners in Lunacy and the round of annual inspections. The result was that, to a great extent, one hospital formed a reflection of the other. The two Berkshire asylums even had an annual cricket match played between them, as noted in *Part One*. Naturally, this was always a home fixture for Broadmoor.

Where Broadmoor departed from Moulsford was in the nature of its referrals. While Moulsford infrequently received petty criminals, all Broadmoor's patients were 'criminal lunatics' sent there by the justice system. These patients were unable to plead or had been found at their trial to be mentally ill, and so they were sentenced to detention 'until Her Majesty's pleasure be known'. Broadmoor dealt also with those who had been declared ill in gaol and were considered dangerous to others.

That judicial element to Broadmoor offers some subtle differences with the life described in *Part One*. The criminal asylum had the same refractory, chronic and convalescent wards, but they were more isolated from each other than the wards at Moulsford, with separate, detached blocks. And while it might be argued that all asylums were constructed to offer an element of public protection, at Broadmoor such protection was part of its reason for existing. A high perimeter wall encircled the site; there were bars on the windows of every room; a higher ratio of staff to patients and much less freedom of movement.

Segregation was also more pronounced, as the women of Broadmoor were kept in their own self-sufficient compound. The chapel was the sole place where both sexes ever shared the same territory, and even then the room was designed so that the women sat in a gallery, behind and above the men. There was no chance of both sides meeting as at chapel and mealtimes at Moulsford. Similarly, there was no coming together at special events, and entertainments and festivals such as Christmas were celebrated by each gender separately.

Broadmoor's size afforded patients a greater variety of spaces: there was a designated quiet reading room, for example, while patients at Moulsford had to make do with whatever library space they could find. There were also more workshops and a more sophisticated system for rewarding work. The Broadmoor patients were paid not just with extra rations, but with money that represented a fraction of the value of the job completed. This money, together with cash gifts from family and friends, was allowed to accrue in a patient's personal account, where it could be used to purchase food and drink, books, magazines or other luxuries delivered from the village or further afield.

Broadmoor additionally offered patients more flexibility with contact from friends and family. This reflected its geographical reach, stretching across not just England and Wales but even the wider British Empire. Visitors to Crowthorne were welcome on any day of the week from Monday to Friday between 10am and noon, and then from 2pm to 4pm. The staff were also prepared to accept visitors at weekends as long as this was arranged in advance. Lodgings would be found in the village for anyone travelling from distance, and the asylum's carriage was used to transport guests. Contrast that with the more restrictive regime at Moulsford, as outlined in *Part One*.

The life of the Broadmoor staff was correspondingly comparable to that of their colleagues in the public system. Many Broadmoor employees joined from other institutions, typically the armed forces or the prison service, and both asylums experienced the same, relatively high turnover of attendants in their early years, before the management gained a better idea of the qualities they sought from applicants. Both asylums also took staff discipline very seriously, and it is here that Broadmoor has made a notable contribution to *Part One*. Within its archive is a short series of 'defaulters' books', which list all the transgressions made by staff. These supplied the story of the two laundry maids who were suspended for 'talking indecently about men', as well as the porter who made a nuisance of himself with the female staff.

Indeed, the defaulters' books suggest that either Broadmoor was party to more staff indiscretions than Moulsford, or the Moulsford superintendents were more inclined to resolve such matters informally. The romance in *Part One* which resulted in pregnancy was between two Broadmoor staff: 24-year-old Arthur Batchelor and 23-year-old Jane Jury. Batchelor resigned on New Year's Day rather than be sacked and Jury joined him after their shotgun marriage; it was perhaps not the start to 1872 that either had envisaged. The married woman who walked home from the station, through the woods with her lover is also a Broadmoor tale, where the woman was the tailor's wife. Her beau was a middle-aged attendant called John Gordon. The day after their illicit promenade Gordon and his own wife Ann were instructed to leave Crowthorne.

It is recommended, then, that if you glimpse these characters as you read this book, to bear in mind that Broadmoor was just another Victorian hospital, albeit a rather special one. It too experienced growth pains throughout the nineteenth century; whereas the Moulsford superintendents bemoaned the workhouses for passing on difficult cases considered beyond treatment, at Broadmoor a similar complaint could be heard against the prisons. Both asylums were largely powerless to resist the demands society made of them.

Chapter 3

The Victorian Asylum: What Happened Next?

By the turn of the twentieth century, the hopeful zeal with which the new public asylums of England and Wales had been embraced had begun to wane. Murmurings of criticism could be heard against asylum culture. It had become apparent throughout the Victorian period that therapeutic motives for asylum care ran in tandem with custodial ones. This was probably inevitable, given the binding of asylums to the machinery of the poor law, and the latter's preference for indoor relief. The poor no longer remained – at greater cost – in their own homes, but were regulated more cheaply in central institutions, and this same logic was applied to pauper lunatics who needed to access the therapy of asylum care.

As the century wore on, the custodial function of asylums was increasingly seen to be the valuable one. Society approved of bringing together patients who were once scattered throughout different towns and villages. The asylum also provided a place to house people for whom it was difficult to find a use, and rather than live independently – or more often, supported by family or employers – these people were drawn together into a single refuge. The result was that the numbers of patients in asylums increased at a disproportionately higher rate than any concurrent increase in the wider population.

Arguments continue about exactly why this was so. There were undoubtedly administrative pressures on the workhouses, which had both financial and management incentives to transfer difficult inmates to the asylum. It also seems plausible that the overcrowding and poor conditions of urban industrialisation had an impact on the concentration of mental illness. What is less easy to demonstrate in the Victorian period is whether the boundaries of madness were pushed wider apart, either by increasing research or the availability of asylum beds. Certainly the medical officers of the public asylum had very little say in admissions, but a greater public awareness of lunacy may have encouraged greater focus on its symptoms.

This increased awareness provides a more troubling explanation for the growth of asylums. It is possible that these new institutions were perceived as offering respite to society, rather than the patients. After all, asylums had been created to look after those who, through no fault of their own, could not help themselves. It was not a great leap to consider that the disabled, the anti-social and the habitually criminal might be better removed from their communities and deposited within an institution where unusual behaviour was guaranteed to find a home. Such an act could also make the local labour more productive, as families no longer had to double work with the demands of challenging friends or family. England's neighbourhoods were given an opportunity to be cleansed of the unable or uncooperative.

This supposition arises from the belief that the asylum formed a natural addition to the prison and the workhouse, becoming part of a triumvirate of great Victorian institutions administering the poor laws. It builds on the knowledge that human traffic also flowed amongst these institutions: the prisons were home to convicts with mental health issues or learning disabilities; while in the workhouses the aged and mentally infirm were tolerated only if they caused no problems. Both these poor-relieving offices flooded the chronic wards at the local asylum.

The hopelessness of many such cases coincided with what would now be described as therapeutic pessimism. Notable commentators, such as Henry Maudsley, contributed unwittingly to the emerging view of the asylum as a human dustbin, somewhere those cast out from society could be shepherded into disciplined exile. Maudsley had a prejudice against asylums, believing them to offer little worthwhile treatment and only limited success; he also believed that many cases of mental illness were incurable, and that to pretend otherwise was a lie. Nor was he alone in this view. In the late nineteenth century, a German doctor called Emile Kraepelin first described the illness later known as schizophrenia, and associated it with an irreversible decline. Kraepelin's work was hugely influential, and his new illness became the crucible in which the concept of the hopeless lunatic patient was forged.

Such was the climate as the Victorian asylum moved into the Edwardian age. Asylums had no longer principally the restorative focus of hope; rather, a small percentage of patients might by chance get well, but the vast majority were expected to do little more than remain sick. Many patients were also social pariahs, exhibiting less the signs of mental illness than some form of personality trait preventing them from being accepted in society. Public asylums were in danger of becoming a dumping ground, and stigma and dehumanisation set into asylum life.

In the first half of the twentieth century this situation became a lot worse. Patient numbers continued to grow and, in keeping with the new-found pessimism, it was decided to siphon off some of the 'hopeless' cases into new institutions. These were created under the Mental Deficiency Act 1913, and built for people with learning disabilities. That Act also made formal divisions between such patients, who were classed as 'idiots', 'imbeciles' or 'feeble-minded' based on intelligence tests and observable factors of self-preservation and improvement. Moulsford, now left only with the 'lunatics', found itself renamed as Berkshire Mental Hospital.

It was a time when eugenics was seriously debated as a way of dealing with mental illness. Winston Churchill argued that those with learning disabilities or personality disorders should be placed in forced labour camps, and a Royal Commission recommended the compulsory sterilisation of patients. This movement reached its natural conclusion with the view that some people may be unworthy of life, a consideration extended to many German patients in the early years of the Second World War.

On the wards at Moulsford, the change of attitude was apparent between the wars. Schizophrenia was suddenly considered to be the most common illness, and the expectation was that any sufferer would spend a lifetime on the chronic wards. Once there, they were looked after by doctors and nurses whose own status in society had risen, while that of their patients had significantly fallen. For the first time, a material gap was visible between the sick and those tending them. Unlike their Victorian counterparts, the nurses of the 1920s and 1930s were positively discouraged from talking to the patients.

The increasing gloom around asylums was only lifted after 1945. The reasons for this were partly social and economic: the post-war boom found employment for many people previously considered surplus, and that group included those whose mental illness affected their capacity for work. These people were now needed, so the wider community gave them a chance to help in whatever way they could. Coincidentally, the employment boom arrived at the same time as the last vestiges of the poor law were swept away. No more were the restrictions of indoor relief to be central to treatment; patients could instead be offered a broader range of care, away from a central institution. The new National Health Service provided services in surgeries and clinics as well as hospitals.

Moulsford joined the NHS in 1948 and was asked to find a new name that would be free of stigma. It chose to become Fair Mile, a suitably anonymous title that turned it into just another institution. This one act of re-branding wiped the asylum off the map, though if the motive was to remove the negative connotations of the Victorian word, the plan was also to restore the Victorian idea of hope. It was part of a rediscovery that patients were people too, and an even greater change in that direction came about in 1959, when the landmark Mental Health Act first gave patients a voice to challenge their detention.

Around the same time, another important development arrived: the prospect of new treatments. For many years, the moral regime had prevailed in public asylums, and the visitor to the ward would have noticed little development from the nineteenth century. The first radical fresh ideas were introduced just before the Second World War, when electro convulsive therapy and insulin comas made their way into public asylums with mixed success. Then, in the late 1950s and early 1960s, modern pharmaceuticals followed, offering if not cures, the alleviation of symptoms and allowing patients to reclaim their former lives. For the clinicians this was a big moment, promising the possibility that most patients could live free of constant care. Vast institutions no longer seemed quite so necessary.

As places like Fair Mile entered a decade of social revolution, the received view of life inside the Victorian asylum was that it too required reappraisal. Living standards outside the asylum had raised immeasurably since Queen Victoria had died, while those inside enjoyed a quality of bed and board unchanged since the turn of the century. In the chronic wards patients had become institutionalised and hopeless, yet new drugs on the admissions wards offered the opportunity of turning even previously static lives around.

It was an era of technical fixes, when prescribing pills was in vogue and the old values of interaction and occupation were generally derided.

It took some time for this shift in medical attitudes to manifest in public policy. Health Minister Enoch Powell had predicted a world free of asylum 'water towers' in 1960, but the gradual move towards discharging long-term patients, begun in the 1950s, continued at a slow pace. When the increase in speed came, it was because the politicians had latched onto a reversal of the old poor law maxim: outdoor relief had now become cheaper to provide than indoor. Asylum buildings were expensive to maintain, as were staff salaries; drugs for out-patients were not. The better option was to dispense with bed and board, to place a welfare payment in one hand and some tablets in the other, and let patients make their own luck instead. Unfortunately, this professional enthusiasm for community-based treatments provided cover for what became savage cuts in mental health services.

The economics of mental health care cannot be dismissed. As the British economy slowed in the 1970s and 1980s, it became harder to discharge people successfully into society. Unemployment became a fact of life for many working people, and those who were already marginalised found a return of hard times. Opportunities for integration shrank, and while the concerted drive to discharge long-term patients continued, it did so without the same results. A new breed of 'revolving door' mental health patient was created, as people found themselves spending shorter, but more regular periods in care. When specialist services were reduced, many patients were admitted to general hospitals instead.

By the time growth improved in the latter 1980s, it had become politically acknowledged that in-patient care was financially undesirable. The preferred option was known as 'care in the community', whereby family and volunteers might provide resources to support the patient alongside the state. This was the moment when the great period of asylum closures was implemented. The end was rapid; nearly forty hospitals shut their doors in the first half of the 1990s and virtually all the Victorian wards were swept away. Fair Mile hung on longer than most, finally discharging its last patient in 2003.

In theory, care in the community could have provided a positive future, where patients were free to make their own choices and were welcomed into society. In some cases this did happen, particularly in the more affluent parts of the country. However, in others, community care offered the risk of what John Talbott, a prominent American psychiatrist, described as replacing 'a single lousy institution with multiple wretched ones'. Studies have estimated that up to 100,000 patients were discharged from Victorian asylums in the second half of the twentieth century. Only 4,000 of those hospital beds were replaced with mattresses in NHS hostels. Other hostels housed the mentally ill who joined the homeless; and where once asylums received patients direct from the prisons and the workhouses, now those patients remain in custody, particularly if they are young; while if they are old, they may be found instead in that most twenty-first century of institutions: the care home.

Mental health services, meanwhile, largely became providers of crisis care. The current NHS offers around 15,000 beds for the mentally ill, and a patient has to present an immediate and serious risk to themselves or others to have a chance of admission. Beds are taken wherever they can be, and it is not unusual for patients to be treated hundreds of miles away from home. Ironically, a modern in-patient ward is full of people who are far more distressed than those who inhabited a Victorian dormitory; the atmosphere is not conducive to respite care. These crisis services have also lost the many peripherals to the old institutions – there have been no systematic replacements for the asylum day-room, its gardens, farm or workshops. Our mental health offer to patients has diminished.

It was not supposed to be this way. Patients were intended to become customers, at liberty to shop around for their health care, with the freedom to consider options rather than to stand alone. But the result has been a social compact far removed from that offered by the Victorians. They guaranteed limited treatment in exchange for your control; we offer whatever you want, but cannot provide it.

This is not to suggest that the Victorian asylums were a panacea. If they were, we would not have wanted other options. In hindsight, though, they failed because our expectations changed. The public asylums were born of a belief that they could be benevolent places, providing a possible cure; they tried to grant a good life for those within them; and even in their darkest days as warehouses, they never meant to be cruel or inhumane.

But we asked too much of them. If they were at fault, it was simply through dealing with the problems that society imposed. Closing the asylums has not brought us any closer to working out how we should respond to mental illness. We still prefer to think that out of mind should mean out of sight.

Chapter 4

Become a Friend of the Victorian Asylum: Researching Archives and Visiting Remaining Sites

Though the great nineteenth century asylums have closed, their presence still looms large in modern memory. Many generations grew up with them and they provide a reference point for debates about mental health care today. They are difficult for medical practitioners or for social historians to ignore.

This book takes a particular approach to the Victorian asylum, striving to note the good intentions behind the institution while also recognising its imperfections. It does not wholeheartedly condemn but attempts to laud the asylum's genuine and heartfelt compassion, even if today we may find such compassion misdirected. I do not pretend that mine is the only valid approach to asylum history. Many people argue passionately that the Victorian asylums were created as merely another instrument of poor law oppression, and that they became places of imprisonment and degradation. Reconciliation with such feelings is not easy.

However if, like me, you do feel that there is something worth commemorating about the Victorian network of public mental health care, then there is good news. For these places have left behind a remarkable, physical legacy, far more so than the other poor law institutions, and this legacy can be glimpsed in virtually every county in the British Isles.

Asylum Buildings

The concrete manifestation of asylum fabric is part of the Victorian contribution to our architectural heritage. Although a number of asylums are no longer standing, they have a far higher survival rate than those other welfare bastions, the workhouses.

This is, in part, due to their very different settings, as workhouses were built typically on the edge of towns and subsequently became surrounded by twentieth century urban sprawl. Most workhouses also joined the NHS as general hospitals and were then converted or replaced as demands required. Yet the asylums were built on those 'airy and healthy situations' that the legislators ordered. These were mostly in parkland and well away from the centres of Victorian population, and post-war redevelopment was not necessary, as there was space enough to build additional structures in the grounds. As a result, not only was an asylum less likely to be altered during its working life, but it was also less likely to fall foul of schemes for town planning after its closure.

The standard of architecture in asylums was invariably far higher than that of workhouses. While the workhouses were designed with a minimum of decoration and adornments, asylum exteriors were almost palatial, as contemporary commentators avowed. Similarly, the workhouse wards had meaner windows, and an absence of the sturdy and spacious interiors praised by the champions of the moral regime. Workhouses reflected their poor law purpose in a way that asylums did not, and this has produced the unforeseen consequence that asylum buildings are more desirable to modern purchasers. Several former Victorian asylums have now been converted into residential use.

In their new form, once public spaces have become private, often gated developments that still keep the outside world out, if perhaps no longer keep the inhabitants shut away. This has been the fate of Fair Mile, which is now a housing project known as Cholsey Meadows. Happily, it has managed to maintain some social housing and community space amongst the 'dramatic, spacious family homes'. You can visit what once was Moulsford and see its restored main block, now largely cleansed of twentieth century infill. You can enter the recreation hall, where the patients once danced to the asylum band, or book the cricket pitch where so many patients played.

Some Victorian asylums are still open as working hospitals. Around ten survived the period of the great closures, including Hanwell – now called St Bernard's Hospital – where John Conolly destroyed every instrument of restraint at the beginning of the Victorian age. The other notable survivor is Broadmoor, though even that will move shortly from its original bricks and mortar to a new hospital next door.

The architecture of Hanwell, Broadmoor and these other grand therapeutic fortresses is still a marvel to behold. Even when derelict they radiate a certain beauty, something that has acquired a cult following amongst those dedicated to abandoned places. Groups of trespassing explorers make it their mission to infiltrate such desolate spaces and take pictures of them. The results are then posted online to illustrate urban decay. It is an unexpected interpretation, and one that is testament to our enduring fascination with asylums.

Asylum Archives

This fascination finds full expression in something even more remarkable than the architectural bequest: the written heritage that these institutions left behind. Here is the phenomenon of asylum archives, a vast resource for the Victorian period, which allows us to see for ourselves, at first-hand, how mental health care developed in our country. Anyone can conduct their own research into these places and the people who lived within them.

We have the Commissioners in Lunacy to thank for this. As well as their rules about ward construction, staff discipline and patient care, the Commissioners produced rules about record-keeping. The result was that recording information was not seen as ephemeral, but as an integral part of life in the Victorian asylum. Every important detail was written into books so that it would not be forgotten.

What the Commissioners could not have predicted is that this paperwork would outlast the institutions that they oversaw, and even the poor laws themselves. The lunacy statutes did not prescribe permanence for asylum records, but, as it has turned out, permanence is the judgement that has been passed on many of them. In part this must be seen as another benefit of those large, sprawling estates, where accumulating records did not necessarily create a storage problem. It was easier to leave them alone than bother to destroy them. In consequence, asylum archives have an even higher survival rate than asylum buildings.

These archives are rarely still on site, but are mostly to be found in the wide network of heritage services run by local councils. Housed once more at the ratepayers' expense, they sit neatly in boxes or on shelves in county repositories, next to other books and papers containing other histories. Lists of them are created and made available to browse. From time to time, members of the public come into the reading room and quote a reference to the staff, whereupon a request is made for the documents to be brought into the light once more.

It is a wonderful thing that so much asylum history is freely available to everyone. There is no requirement for visitors to be learned scholars, and only a little acclimatisation is necessary to decipher the arcane language and unfamiliar handwriting. Persevere and you will be able to unwrap the stories of the past neatly packaged up inside the records. The stories within are very powerful, and every individual has a tale to tell.

That tale begins first in Victorian society, before it draws you into the asylum and its routine. In an asylum archive you can seek out the documents created by the justices and the medical officers – the admissions registers and case books, monthly minutes and annual reports, wages books and ledgers.

While researching this book I drew on various management records from the senior men (and they always were men) at Moulsford and Broadmoor. The superintendent's annual reports to his committee, which are augmented with a dazzling array of what might loosely be termed performance statistics, provide an insight into not just the regime but also its motives. Superintendents' characters betray themselves as they write these summaries, and the same is true for their monthly reports or journals, while the committee minute books provide the key source for decision-making. Thus a picture of day-to-day life emerges and you can begin to place the people of the asylum within it.

Those people existed on two sides of a practical divide. The staff, though they were closely tied to their work, were not confined as the patients were. Neither was their employment subjected to observation and note-taking. The asylum's main record-keeping interest in its employees was twofold: in paying their wages, and punishing their misdemeanours. *Part One* of this book made use of wages books to list employees, while rules, orders and disciplinary records illustrated how staff were expected to behave. No life stories are to be found here, but there are anecdotes and incidents aplenty.

The other side of the divide is well catered for with source material. Patient records were the main focus of the Commissioners' guidance. I find these records very humbling, as within them is proof of the omnipresence of mental illness in any society at any time. Here are people who are no longer in control of their own lives, the responsibility for which is given over to someone else. The records are a cenotaph for those buried deep within them; an undeclared monument for thousands of Victorian people.

For me this is probably the most interesting facet of asylum archives. It is very rare to find in one source so much about the life of the ordinary person. These patients did not possess swathes of land or titles, they did not hold high office; they worked as so many of us do in offices, factories or farms, or else they raised families – as husbands, wives, fathers, mothers. Theirs are the voices that history finds it easiest to ignore, and yet if you look within the records of a public asylum you will find so many of them.

Patients' names are listed in the registers of admission and the registers of discharges, removals and deaths. Names, ages, places of abode and occupation are recorded alongside the dates of their asylum stay. This is where you first try to find a patient and their identifying number. From here, if you are lucky, you may be able to go elsewhere to discover more beyond the barest comings and goings. All asylums kept series of casebooks and case files, which reflect the distinction made between the administrative papers for each patient and the medical observations carried out during their stay.

To call the case files an administrative bundle is perhaps an injustice. Although they include the necessary paperwork that authorised detention, they might also feature correspondence from family or friends or even from the patient, and they are by no means as dry as the title might suggest. For Broadmoor, these files are often the only place to find the patient's own voice. Frustratingly, a filing cabinet full of Moulsford's papers was lost to the skip shortly before the other archives could be secured.

Happily, within a metal bookcase near the old committee room at Moulsford were almost all the asylum's casebooks, from the very first through to the 1920s. When the bookcase doors were opened several rows of white spines peered out, as polished and as smooth as the bones of any skeleton. In gold leaf capitals, each one proclaims 'Male' or 'Female' with a volume number. Every page is headed by a patient's name, an age – *aet*, in abbreviated medical Latin – and the date of admission. Beneath are the notes, written up by the asylum's junior doctor.

After the initial listing of 'factors indicating insanity' on admission, there is a description of the patient's mental and physical states. 'Answers reluctantly and in a very low voice'; 'conversation is incoherent and utterly senseless'; 'markedly deficient in knowledge of even the most ordinary and common things'; such were the verdicts meted out on Moulsford's new arrivals. Beneath that description come further notes, added weekly at first and then monthly or quarterly. These notes show the patient's progress through the system.

The notes often tell of stasis; 'No change' is a common refrain, with 'bodily health fair, still irrational' a slight variation. Such notes add credence to the suggestion that patients ended up forgotten, on the chronic wards for decades. If any recovery was under way, then there was a chance that no one ever noticed. However, to dismiss the notes as unenlightening would be to do them a disservice. They include details of outbursts or accidents and also describe delusions or fears. They amplify each case, giving you a sense of whether a patient was at peace with themselves or perpetually troubled, angry or resigned.

Each time I browse one of the Moulsford or Broadmoor records I am distracted by someone new, whom I have not met before. I want to find out about them and to try and understand them. I feel that I ought to rescue them from obscurity because their stories should be heard, but perhaps I am simply projecting a new paternalism on to these patients; one that is just as judgemental as anything the Victorians offered. Like James Murdoch, I believe that I am labouring for my fellows.

If so, then I am not alone. In celebrating the people who spent time in the Victorian asylum, the truth is that I have arrived somewhat late upon the scene. For while we argue over the benefits of the residential home or the benefits of community care, while we debate the stigma that is attached to mental illness, an entirely unexpected challenge to our stereotypes has come about through the efforts of Britain's large band of family historians. They have taken up asylum archives without a thought for the politics of the institution.

Every day, up and down the country, these personal detectives search excitedly for ancestors whose names they have found secreted in the records of asylum care, wishing to add them to their lists of forebears. Extensive access to historic resources like the census has opened up the remnants of Victorian communities previously hidden to all but the most dedicated researcher. Anyone can look for names of patients and then find out more about them. So people do. After a century as outcasts, a quiet revolution of rehabilitation is currently at hand, as many unknown pauper lunatics have their graves marked by genealogists and their experience resurrected.

There is something that we can all learn from this. Like the patients before them, family historians are mostly ordinary men and women from across the walks of life. They have no received knowledge about the asylum, they pursue no set agenda. In the absence of these encumbrances, they have sought out those moonstruck souls who form part of their flesh and blood; more than that, they have embraced them willingly and without prejudice, crafting a supportive branch for them onto many a family tree.

So here are the true friends of the Victorian asylum. The heirs of patients have brought us back to the values of William Tuke and the Retreat, back to the virtues of moral treatment. Those who suffer from mental illness are only people just like all of us. We treat them no differently to anyone else. We respect them, we value them and we join with them. We spent the past together, and we go forward together.

Chapter 5

Before You Go: Moulsford Patient Portraits

One thing that this book has not been able to do is dwell in depth on the life stories of individual Moulsford patients. The hero of a tale entitled 'Life in the Victorian Asylum' has to be the institution, rather than the people within it and so, although patients often appear in the preceding chapters, they are principally defined by their illness.

Nonetheless, that illness is only a part of their story, and it does not reflect the fact that every patient also had a life outside the asylum. They were not solely mental health patients; they were everyday Victorian people whose misfortune was simply to fall sick at some point during their lives.

In this spirit, here are some brief pen portraits of Moulsford patients. Each was a real person. England's county asylum network was set up to treat people like them.

John James Lee, John Runciman and Duncan McPhee

The public asylum was obliged to take any patient in its catchment who required relief. They were usually local people who had lived in the area all their lives, but not entirely: anyone who could establish (or have established for them) a legal right of settlement, or who simply could not be allocated to another poor law union, might end up falling onto the accounts of the ratepayers. The result is that various tramps and travellers can be found in the Moulsford admissions registers.

These travellers were often attracted by some local feature that drew in residents from further afield – agricultural work, fairs, army camps – but they could also be inspired to travel by their illness. In Berkshire, the royal residence at Windsor Castle was an attraction for lunatics who had incorporated the monarchy into their delusions. Over the years a handful were admitted to Moulsford; though what makes John James Lee, John

Runciman and Duncan McPhee stand out is that they all decided to make the journey within a few months of each other in 1877.

John James Lee was a wealthy timber merchant from Bury St Edmunds, who arrived in Windsor by train that spring. He walked through the town to the Castle gate, ran straight through it and was picked up in the quadrangle by a suspicious constable, who had witnessed Lee's hasty dash and went in pursuit of him. Under questioning, Lee iterated his descent from the house of Stuart and said he had been twice married to Queen Victoria. After a few weeks in Moulsford he was removed to the Ipswich Asylum and ended up in a private madhouse, close to his wife and children, where he died in 1910.

McPhee and Runciman had trekked even further. They both believed that they had important messages to deliver to the Queen. Runciman, a short young man with jet black hair and dark eyes, was an Edinburgh carpenter who had quit his job and then walked all the way to Balmoral. Having been turned away, he took the train south to Windsor, whereupon he was arrested at the Castle gate, taken first to the workhouse and then onto Moulsford. His fate was similar to Lee's: the asylum medical officers made contact with Runciman's father and he was discharged to the Royal Edinburgh Asylum on the same day that Lee went back to Suffolk.

McPhee faired slightly differently. A pale, fair-haired Scot, he was a 36-year-old, highly educated law clerk, who had also left his employment to pursue an unusual fantasy. McPhee believed he had uncovered a Jesuit plot to destroy the Protestant religion and agents of that league had begun to put poison in his food. McPhee then became convinced that the Jesuits had moved to persecute his friends, so he avowed to tell the monarch of the plot before any more people came to harm.

Like Runciman, McPhee started his odyssey at Balmoral, then camped out near Buckingham Palace and Osborne House, before eventually arriving in Windsor. He presented himself at the Castle and stated his intention both to warn the Queen of a conspiracy and also to marry Princess Beatrice. He was immediately placed in custody. Yet, unlike his fellow countryman, McPhee arrived at the asylum without any information about his friends or family, and no attempt was made to send him home.

McPhee's fate was to stay at Moulsford. His was a classic case of monomania. McPhee could hold an intelligent conversation on many subjects, but if the topic moved towards religion then his illness showed itself. He comes across in his notes as an unhappy man. Though he was put to work in the asylum garden – a convalescing task – and helped the clerk with his office duties, McPhee's constant paranoia about the Jesuits made him troublesome and sometimes violent. On occasions he refused his food and was force-fed with the pump. He also expressed his disapproval of the asylum's entertainments, refusing to help write the programmes for events, and once standing up mid-performance to castigate the staff for the earthy humour of their songs.

Perhaps due to his greater education, McPhee never quite fitted in with the other patients. 'Fond of showing his superiority of language and thoughts' was one note; 'wishes to regulate the arrangement of the asylum' was another. He continued to believe that his food was poisoned, while he also developed the fear that electricity was used to torture him. He claimed that Dr Gilland kept an iron instrument under his patients' beds through which currents could be passed.

McPhee was in Moulsford for nine years. He had contracted tuberculosis before his admission and the disease eventually killed him in 1886.

Thomas Ashton

As I have previously hinted, a proportion of public asylum patients had some sort of military background. The percentages in Moulsford were not as high as in Broadmoor – where approximately one in ten of the early male patients had served in the forces – but ex-soldiers were a persistent feature in the annual admissions tables.

Thomas Ashton was one of these. He was born in 1833 in Huddersfield. As a teenager he moved to Dublin and subsequently enlisted in the army. He served for fifteen years, mostly in the Royal Scots Greys. Ashton cannot have been an easy colleague: he was branded with the letters 'B C' (meaning of 'Bad Character') on his chest, before he was given a dishonourable discharge. The army clearly had a point, because shortly after he left his regiment Ashton was picked up in Oxford for attempting to pass on stolen goods. In January 1867 he was convicted in Abingdon and given six months' hard labour in Reading Gaol.

While he was in gaol Ashton's excitable behaviour caught the attention of the medical officer. He was certified as suffering from mental illness, classified as a criminal lunatic and admitted to Littlemore Asylum. He was also boarded out at Fisherton House in Salisbury, then brought back to Berkshire as one of the first men transferred to Moulsford when it opened.

Ashton was diagnosed by Dr Gilland and his team as suffering from mania. He was an elated character who believed himself to have been blessed with superhuman skills, a champion prize fighter and the cleverest man in the world, capable of earning one pound every minute. His constant chatter sounded very positive, though his mood in the asylum was somewhat bullying, and he alternated between extreme courtesy and outright abuse.

Like Broadmoor, Moulsford also found that the convicted criminals were the patients who were prone to escape. Ashton fitted this description and he became something of a serial escaper, though none of his attempts were very successful. During his first in 1874, he ran away while he was supposed to be cleaning corridors. He reached a house in North Moreton, where a friend of his lived, but he was less welcome than he had anticipated and ended up detained while help was sent for.

The following year he made off from an airing court, intending to walk along the railway line from Moulsford to London. On that occasion he made it as far as the adjacent bridge over the Thames, then spotted the Beetle and Wedge Inn and decided to stop for a pint. The landlord sent a messenger up the road for help. In 1880, Ashton ran away during a game of cricket and was retrieved from the nearby town of Wallingford. His last foray came in 1885, when he simply walked across the asylum fields, first to the main road and then a further six miles across the Berkshire Downs, where he was spotted at the railway station in the village of Compton.

Despite this tendency, Ashton became something of a reformed character at Moulsford. Though he continued to shout and curse, his sporting prowess was indeed marked and he excelled at tennis and at cricket, becoming the institution's finest fast bowler (for which he received a brief mention in *Part One*). This did not help with his delusions of grandeur: 'still the most conceited man in the asylum' read one exasperated note. Ashton was also a dedicated worker. A big, burly man, for years he helped out chopping logs for firewood (which might have been thought a risky move) and also cleaning his ward. He was noted for the exceptionally high standards he brought to his work.

This was the contradiction in Ashton: at times intimidating and threatening, he spared no effort at making sure all was in order around him. He was known to care deeply for the wellbeing of his fellow patients; when he became severely ill with diarrhoea in 1883 he simply took himself off to the billiard room to avoid bothering anyone else. Realising that he was settled, the staff left him there to follow a diet of milk and opium until he recovered. Shortly afterwards, Ashton gained his highest asylum accolade when he was appointed as a volunteer nurse to the sick. The gentle giant spent many hours in the Moulsford infirmary caring for his fellow patients. When he died in 1906 superintendent James Murdoch attended his funeral.

Emily Parham

Emily Parham's story is one that is repeated many times throughout the Moulsford records: that of a young mother in need of help. What makes Emily's tale a suitable one on which to close is because she links the two asylums whose histories have informed this book. Hers is a Broadmoor story as well as a Moulsford one.

She was born Emily Deller, the daughter of a carter, in Shoreditch in 1840. After working for some years in a London goods office, in her late twenties Emily joined the staff at Broadmoor as a seamstress. It was here that she met Henry Parham, the asylum's Sussex-born stableman. The two courted, and with the permission of the asylum authorities they wed in 1871, before moving into married quarters on the Crowthorne estate.

Emily quickly fell pregnant, but seven months into her term she began to exhibit unusual behaviour. She was feverish in manner, rambling in conversation, and she believed that she had been possessed by the devil, who was attempting to influence her with destructive thoughts. For two months Henry nursed her at home until the baby was born: a daughter, also called Emily. There was a brief period of respite when Emily nursed her child, yet before long her delusions returned with a vengeance. She started breaking things around the house and then threatened to kill herself and the baby.

Broadmoor's medical officers stepped in. Their asylum was home to many mothers who had murdered their children, and they did not wish to receive another from amongst their own community. David Cassidy, Broadmoor's deputy superintendent, spoke at length to Henry Parham before the doctor signed the form required to admit Emily to Moulsford. She arrived on the female wards in November 1872.

Shortly afterwards her baby grew sick, and Henry fought desperately to save his daughter to no avail. She died at home. Henry was now in married quarters on his own, while his wife remained at Moulsford, where she suffered a fit so severe that it left her screaming, convulsing and bedridden. Her health continued to decline until she too died in October 1874, aged 34. Her death certificate records the cause as 'general paralysis of the insane': which we now know was syphilis, and this infection may have also accounted for the death of her child.

Devastated, Henry Parham resigned from Broadmoor and moved to Reading, where he looked after the horses at a brewery. A few years later he took a new wife, Annie, and they went on to have nine children together. When his work as a stableman dried up, Henry became a house painter, and soon after, the now elderly couple moved back to Crowthorne. For the last twenty years of his life Henry lived once more within a half-hour walk of Broadmoor. He died in 1921 at the grand old age of 80.

Emily's short life illustrates the sudden change in fortunes that a crisis can bring about; Henry's rather longer span illustrates the choices facing families of asylum patients. After his young wife was removed from him, Henry had no option but to make the best he could of the situation. If Emily had not died so young, Henry would have joined the pool of visitors who came month after month, year after year to Moulsford to sit in the panelled waiting room, staring at the printed regulations while their partners were fetched from the wards. In many ways, the lives of those visitors were just as static as those of the patients. Chronic illness was – and remains – the cruellest sentence.

Sources

The Broadmoor and Fair Mile Archives

I am very fortunate to look after two Victorian mental health archives in my day job, and both of these have been invaluable sources in the writing of this book.

The Berkshire Record Office took custody of the Broadmoor archive in 2004. My book *Broadmoor Revealed* is based on its contents and how they can be used. For *Life in the Victorian Asylum*, more information came from the Broadmoor management and staff records. Of particular interest were the Victorian annual reports (Berkshire Record Office reference D/H14/A2/1/1/1-13), Council of Supervision minutes (D/H14/A1/2/1-3) and Commissioners in Lunacy reports (D/H14/A1/1/1/1-2), as well as staff instructions (D/H14/B1/2/2/1), order books (D/H14/A2/1/5/1, A2/1/7/1) and defaulters books (D/H14/B1/3/1/1-3).

The Fair Mile archive came into the Berkshire Record Office during 2001 and 2002, just before the hospital closed. Fair Mile, in its guise as the Moulsford Asylum, has provided the bulk of the archive material that has inspired this book.

There are various relevant collections to point you towards in Berkshire Record Office. There are annual reports to the justices (Q/AL12/1-5) and monthly reports to the Committee of Visitors (D/H10/A4/1-7). The patient casebooks, from which much of the anecdotal case details comes, are in two series for males (D/H10/D2/1/1-13) and females (D/H10/D2/2/1-17). There is also a series of chaplain's journals for the period (D/H10/E1/1-6).

Although a number of real patients are named in the book, for the handful of cases in the *Diagnosis* chapter I have used initials in order to preserve the anonymity of patients within the Victorian asylum. I can dispense with this conceit here, and list them by their full names:

- E.B.: Ellen Brookes, housewife, from East Hagbourne, admitted to Moulsford in 1887
- J.T.: James Turvey, schoolmaster, from Windsor, admitted in 1871
- J.B.: Julia Batten, field labourer, from Newbury, admitted in 1878
- J.N.: James Neville, labourer, from Reading, admitted in 1870
- S.J.A.: Sarah Jane Allott, dressmaker, from Reading, admitted in 1879
- J.H.: Jesse Horn, ex-soldier, from Englefield, admitted in 1870
- W.S.: William Shanks, blacksmith, from Cookham, admitted in 1874
- H.T.: Hesther Turrill, housewife, from Reading, admitted in 1875
- S.C.: Sarah Cannon, cellarman's wife, from Maidenhead, admitted in 1871
- F.S.: Frederick Simmonds, ex-soldier, from Reading, admitted in 1874
- F.B.: Frederick Benning, from Binfield, admitted in 1872 [Benning subsequently ended up in Broadmoor where his BRO file reference is D/H14/D2/2/1/785]
- A.H.: Agnes Harrow, housewife, from Reading, admitted in 1880
- J.Hr.: James Hester, policeman, from London but charged to the Faringdon Union, admitted in 1871
- J.Ht.: John Hewett, unemployed, from Wellington in Somerset, admitted in 1880

Similarly, four anonymous patients have a brief mention in the *Discharge* chapter. They are:

- W.G.: William Goddard, carpenter, from Leckhampstead, admitted to Moulsford in 1878
- F.T.: Frederick Todd, house painter, from Windsor, admitted in 1878
- E.F.: Eliza Fullbrook, baker, from Reading, admitted in 1878
- J.Bo.: Jane Bowyer, servant, from Easthampstead, admitted in 1878

Another patient crops up on three occasions in *Part One* but is never named. Selina Lambourne was admitted in 1893, via the Berkshire Assizes, where she had been charged with attempted suicide. It was Selina who was fond of swallowing hair pins. Happily, she spent only nine months in Moulsford before being discharged to the care of her family in Kent.

There are, of course, many other asylum archives up and down the country. I have been lucky enough to have insight from the archives of Brookwood (Surrey), Fisherton House (Wiltshire), Littlemore (Oxfordshire) and Rainhill (Liverpool), but I will let you hunt out your own local ones, as that is part of the fun of research.

Bibliography

Books and Other Printed Sources

A handful of contemporary Victorian texts were essential companions during my research:

Bucknill, John Charles; Tuke, Daniel Hack, *A Manual of Psychological Medicine*, J & A Churchill, (1879 edition).

Commissioners in Lunacy, *Suggestions and instructions with reference to site: general arrangement of buildings: construction of buildings: plans and particular: estimates: of lunatic asylums*, HMSO, (1871).

Medico-Psychological Association, Newington, H H (ed), *Handbook for Attendants on the Insane*, Bailliére, Tindall and Cox, (1899 edition).

Mercier, Charles, *Lunatic Asylums: Their Organisation and Management*, Charles Griffin and Co Ltd, (1894).

I have also used some of the printed annual Commissioners in Lunacy reports, which give a running commentary on the development of asylums during most of the nineteenth century. The Lunacy Acts and County Asylum Acts were also of help.

Local newspapers are an invaluable source for making sense of the more sensational events in local asylums. Coroners inquests, trials and festivals are often reported in some detail and in diary form, without the journalistic interventions in modern media. The *Reading Mercury* was my paper of choice for this book, with the *Berkshire Chronicle* second. Both these resources can be found in Reading Library.

I tried to read as few contemporary sources as possible while I was writing this book, because I wanted to react solely to the Victorian take on asylum care. However, many books and articles have been written about the Victorian approach to mental health and the following are recent books that I have drawn on while writing *Life in the Victorian Asylum*. They all provide more extensive bibliographies for further reading than I will attempt here:

Arnold, Catharine, *Bedlam: London and its Mad*, Simon and Schuster, (2008).

Barham, Peter, *Closing the Asylum*, Penguin, (1992).

Porter, Roy, *Madness: A Brief History*, Oxford University Press, (2002).

Rutherford, Sarah, *The Victorian Asylum*, Shire Books, (2008).

Wise, Sarah, *Inconvenient People: Lunacy, Liberty and the Mad-doctors in Victorian England*, Bodley Head, (2012).

Index